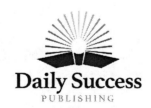

OTHER BOOKS BY DAYNA STEELE

Havana: 101 Ways to Rock Your World

In the Classroom: 101 Ways to Rock Your World

Welcome to College! 101 Ways to Rock Your World

On the Golf Course: 101 Ways to Rock Your World

101 Ways to Rock Your World: Everyday Activities for Success Every Day

Rock to the Top: What I Learned about Success from the World's
Greatest Rock Stars

SURVIVING ALZHEIMER'S

WITH FRIENDS, FACEBOOK, AND A REALLY BIG GLASS OF WINE

Why A Book Of Facebook Posts?

I TRULY NEVER grasped what "The Long Goodbye" meant until you started these updates.

Your updates have made me laugh and cry but mostly to realize that I am not alone in the journey.

I hope that you write and publish a book about your journey. It will be so helpful to others beginning this roller-coaster ride. The good and the bad, it is all so informative. Laughter and tears!

What I've learned from your posts helped me help an older friend whose husband is suffering from dementia. She described some of the hell she's going through which is compounded by the fact she's an "old-fashioned kind of girl" who finds it very stressful to challenge her husband. I recalled some of your posts about getting to the doctor even when your mom did not want to go. I shared that and she is going to try some of the same techniques with him. You are casting pebbles into the pond and the ripples are not yet finished spreading.

Sharing your moments with your mom is helping so many who either fear this awful issue or are caretakers currently. I am reading everything I can to find a way I can help families living this.

Your honesty is so refreshing.

Do you know how many people you would touch with a book? I think your story is the story of many. I have never heard it told in such detail. Most people try to hold it together, but won't share it with friends.

I think it's very brave and generous of you to share these reports instead of sweeping the whole situation under the rug. Many of us have already gone through this; and many others may soon have to face it with their own parents. At least they will have your lead to follow and a reference point to understand what to expect.

These updates have empowered those that may someday have to face the same thing.

I hope you are considering writing a book with all this vast knowledge. As painful as it may seem, it would be such a blessing to those that will inevitably follow in your footsteps — it will be therapeutic for them as you say it is for you.

Reading your experience helps but scares me too! It's not for wimps. Hugs.

I am so grateful for your posts. Your "ministry" brings much strength and comfort to many and I hope to you as well.

The way you deal with this and share it, including the humor you find, must be a big help to others going through the same journey.

Thank you for sharing the "real side" of Alzheimer's.

These posts are beyond educational.

Thank you so much for sharing the journey you are taking with your mom during the devastating illness. The sharing of your feelings and your mom's journey are some of the best support I have found.

This is incredible. Gives me such insight into what my mother was going through.

I am learning so much from you. You have to write a book about this. Your observations are so gripping and so graphic I can't imagine. There is a tremendous market for this information. Please share it.

I know this must be painful, but it is helpful to help us prepare for my parents in the near future.

You really should put all these posts together and write a book someday, the way you write makes you a perfect storyteller, with your human touch and the brutal honesty, good, bad and other wise, no telling how many people you have already helped and how many more would get so much out of you sharing this part of your mother's and your lives.

Bravo to you for your honesty, and also for educating people.

Please continue your posts. It is important to know the things you are going through. Alzheimer's is a disease that many people are not familiar with and this gives all of us an idea of what is expected and how it can be handled. Thank you so much.

Only someone who has walked this path understands all the emotions.

I wish someone had shared his or her journey as you are now, so it would have helped prepare me for what to expect.

We can see what may be coming our way and are better prepared, thanks to you blazing the trail for us.

Thank you for sharing publicly — we often feel so alone.

This is an important window to a disease that scares many — so much so we don't want to think it's really so terrible. It's terrible.

SURVIVING ALZHEIMER'S

WITH FRIENDS, FACEBOOK, AND A REALLY BIG GLASS OF WINE

A CAREGIVER'S GUIDE TO LOVE, HUMOR, PATIENCE, CONFUSION, ANGER, AND WINE

Dayna Steele
with Heather Rossiello

DAILY SUCCESS PUBLISHING
USA

ISBN-13: 9781519370846
ISBN-10: 1519370849

Large quantity purchases of this book are available at a discount. Contact:
www.yourdailysuccesstip.com
info@yourdailysuccesstip.com

Printed in the United States of America
Publish date: March 2016
Front cover photo by Jeremy Pierson and designed by Tracy Spiess

To my wonderful mother Fran Nicholson.
- Dayna

To Mike, Sam, and Kate for encouraging me.
- Heather

CONTENTS

Americans whisper the word 'Alzheimer's' because their government whispers the word 'Alzheimer's,' and although a whisper is better than silence that the Alzheimer's community has been facing for decades, it's still not enough. It needs to be yelled and screamed to the point that it finally gets the attention and the funding that it deserves and needs.

- Seth Rogen, in his address to Congress, February 26, 2014

Opening Words: Dayna Steele

Paragraphs so marked originally published in the Houston Chronicle "Gray Matters" August 25, 2015

ODDS ARE YOU picked up this book because you are caring for someone with Alzheimer's, have your suspicions about a loved one, or may be concerned about yourself. That is no surprise. The statistics are staggering and growing. Or maybe you got the book because you have followed this journey on my Facebook page. That is where I have lived it out the last few years.

This book isn't to make you feel sorry for Mom, my family, or for me. It is to give you permission to live and laugh and love and cry and throw things no matter where you are in your journey with Alzheimer's. This book is to tell you don't worry, there is no right way or wrong way to approach this crazy-ass disease — you just get through it the best you can.

My Facebook Alzheimer's update posts, from the time Dad died until we lost Mom, became a personal journey of coping with Alzheimer's on a very public forum. It was cathartic for me — once I wrote the post, I let go of the sadness, tears, anger, or hate, whatever I was feeling and moved on — never realizing how much the posts would help others, and me.

Since early 2013, I have been chronicling Fran Nicholson's journey through Alzheimer's on my Facebook page. Fran is my mom, so this is my *journey as well. The posts started as a way to let family and close friends know what was happening, so I didn't have to repeat the details over and over. It was hard enough to say it once: Mom has been diagnosed with Alzheimer's. You try it. Now say it 100 times, and see how happy you are.**

Caregivers need a support system, family, and/or friends, to help you through the process. You will be dragged deep into sadness and depression. You will be confused and worried as to whether you are doing things correctly. You will be worn out from all the effort it takes — whether you take care of your loved one in your own home or in a care facility. It will take an emotional and physical toll on you no matter what your circumstances are like nothing else ever has. You will feel like you are losing a loved one over and over and over as the disease progresses. When it's all over, you will be stunned at the depth of grief even though you knew it was coming and have grieved through the entire process. You'll rack your brain with guilt, all the what-ifs. And, it will be somewhat strange to all of a sudden have so many extra hours in a day.

Having always been a fan of dark humor, I used it to relieve some of the tears and fears. I figured if something made me laugh out loud, perhaps others would see the funny side of such an unfunny adventure.*

There is one thing I did not mention in all the updates but felt it needed to be mentioned in this book. More often than not, it is one family member or friend who does most of the caregiving and coordinating. Other family members and friends live far away or are in denial and far away from accepting what is happening.

My mother's brother and wife, my wonderful uncle and aunt, stepped right in to help and do as much as they could. In the beginning, my only sibling was going through his own crisis with an impending divorce and lived on the other side of town. Another relative commented that Mom was probably 'faking it for attention'. I can't remember one person from my late father's side of the family coming to see her. And, as time progressed, even Mom's closest friends stopped calling and visiting.

As the disease has progressed, the humor subsided and stark crept in. The posts grew more personal, more raw. I just had to let it out. And I did. Then a strange thing started to happen. It was no longer family and close friends following along — it was friends of friends, former KLOL fans (I used to be a deejay), and complete strangers asking to be Facebook friends or at least follow along. We became a support community for each other.*

There were times I was so angry that none of them were more involved or at least more sympathetic to what was happening. It was my teenage son who helped me let go of that anger by pointing out if my immediate family and mom's friends accepted the seriousness and the level of the problem, they would then have to be a part of the heart-wrenching solution. They just weren't in a position or frame of mind to do that at the time. It became my journey they joined from a far. I must add that my brother did finally accept the inevitable and became my hero; talking me off the ledge at various times, letting me rant, letting me cry as well as taking over and giving me a break so many times.

Stories like those add up fast and can be crushing to your soul. About mid-2014 it began to dawn on me that I was writing these updates, and posting them on Facebook, as a way of letting go. I didn't need therapy; I just needed a keyboard and Facebook. Once I shared whatever was happening, bad or awful, it was if I had released it into the Universe. I no longer had to carry around that piece of dark luggage.*

Until that happened though, I needed support. My Wonder Husband and sons were amazing but it was equally hard on them and they could only do so much to help me — emotionally or physically. That first year we realized something was wrong, I found the more I shared on

Facebook, the more cathartic it became for me. Facebook acquaintances and total strangers filled in the void my family and mom's friends were not filling for me.

I shared what I found to be hysterical dark humor and found others had just as funny, if not funnier stories, as well. Occasionally, I shared the sad and you rallied around me. When I had a question, you had the answers. And, you posted articles, information, your own stories, and messages of support, pictures, and videos on a daily basis to keep me going. There wasn't space in this book to share the thousands of comments made on my Facebook posts but please know I read each and every one, sometimes twice or more.

> *There have been those, the naysayers, who chastise me for being so honest, so open, and at times so crass, for exposing my mom and her decline so publicly. This sharing is for me. This sharing is for Mom. This is for you who may have found yourself on this journey. Or will. Talk about it. Write about it. Let it out or it will eat you alive.**

My friend Peter Shankman once said figure out what your demons are and find a way to work through them without succumbing to the dark side. My demon has been this insidious disease known as Alzheimer's and you, my dear Facebook friend, have kept me from the dark side.

Dayna Steele is the creator and CEO of YourDailySuccessTip.com. She is the author of Rock to the Top: What I Learned about Success from the World's Greatest Rock Stars, *the creator of the* 101 Ways to Rock Your World *book series, a Rock Radio Hall of Famer, and a successful entrepreneur. A professional business speaker, Dayna is also a regular contributor to Fox News Houston, consults Fortune 500 companies, and is married to author Charles Justiz. Her mom, Fran Nicholson, was her biggest fan.*

Opening Words: Heather Rossiello

I STARTED THIS journey with Dayna Steele in November of 2012. A simple meeting that I had no idea would lead us to this book project together. I had messaged her on Facebook asking her to meet with me and sign copies of her book "101 Ways to Rock Your World" as Christmas gifts for the social workers I worked with. I had admired her during her radio days and loved her books as well.

On that day in November Dayna was making one of life's most difficult decisions. I had no idea that I would be a sounding board and become a part of her journey with her through her mother's Alzheimer's.

The decision she was making that day was to tell her mom that she must move into an Assisted living facility next door to the nursing home that her father already resided in. Her mother could no longer be so far from Dayna or take complete care of herself. This would allow Dayna to visit and facilitate both her mother and father's needs more easily.

It was a tough parental decision but that is what we do become as our parents move into those later elderly years. We become the parents. We become the boss of most of their day-to-day living decisions. And as Dayna has experienced some of these decisions are much more difficult than others.

She soon would lose her father and her mother's care and condition would take her on a path that she had absolutely no knowledge or experience with, so in that journey she made the conscious decision to begin a new education so that she could be the best support to her mother as possible, through knowledge, love, and understanding, Facebook and a lot of wine … she brought her Facebook readers into her personal experience with her mom and Alzheimer's.

This brought me into her world further, still not knowing that I would be a support to her in taking Dayna's Facebook data and photos and bringing it to life for the world to read and become more educated and understanding of those that suffer this horrible disease called Alzheimer's. It also gave caregivers a place to voice and vent their day-to-day experiences or history of experience with those they cared for and loved with dementia or Alzheimer's.

I had no idea the evolution this experience would create in my own personal life on every level imaginable. I would learn to look at life and myself through a completely new pair of glasses, having been some level of caregiver most of my life, I now respect that job with such gratitude. I have learned what it means to truly love your parent even in the very most difficult of times and how family, good friends, social media and a little wine can get us through just about anything.

Heather Rossiello has spent a majority of her adult life in the real estate industry and raising two kids now in college. She has also headed numerous committees and worked on community projects for various local schools and non-profit organizations, most recently working with Special Needs Children in her local school district.

Acknowledgements

First and foremost, thanks to Mark Zuckerberg for inventing Facebook.

To my wonder husband Charlie and my sons for wiping up the buckets of tears and pouring the wine. To Uncle Jim and Aunt Mary Gilmore for providing and helping drink the wine and taking care of Mom.

To my brother Scooter Nicholson and my nieces Lorelle and Madison for their love and help.

To friend and editor Linda Lee who made this trip with her mom before me and provided a road map and wine. To Melissa Stevens who went there before me as well and was always available for a phone call and wine. To cousin Kay Jenkins for the support, really big wine glasses, and wine. To Cheryl Evans and Mija for all the dog love and wine. To Doris and Roy Hood for carpooling elderly parents and wine.

To Mom's partner in crime Bonnie Schoellkopf who was there to be her friend when I could not be there. To Monica Golden at CVS who made picking up prescriptions always a nice visit with a friend. To Eylat Poliner who helped me begin this book.

To the *Houston Chronicle's* Lisa Gray whose comments encouraged me to go forward with the book.

To Tracy Spiess for coming out of retirement to design the book cover. I don't know how I could do a book without you. You inspire me.

To everyone who took the time to go by and see Mom even if it was just once or only for a few minutes. Those visits were like solid gold to her. Same to those who sent cards, letters, and gifts. She loved mail until the end.

To Heather Rossiello for asking if she could be of any help with this book project. Hands down, the book never would have been written or finished without her. And, to Heather's sweet family for letting me borrow her for a while.

To Carla Medlenka who discovered all of the incorrect "Moms" and "moms." We hope we corrected most of them, however, we decided to keep the Facebook posts and comments as they were originally written. That and Mom was always worth a capital "M" to me.

And, to each and every Steeleworker who traveled this journey with me on Facebook — I like you.

If you can laugh at it, you can deal with it.
- Joan Rivers

2013:

HOUSTON WE HAVE A PROBLEM

JANUARY 12, 2013

Surprise limo and champagne for Mom in Las Vegas. May have to take her to Chippendales!

That's what it's all about!

You're in Vegas? (Dayna's husband)

Dayna note: Mom loved to gamble; she and Dad would take trips all the time to Louisiana to play the slots. Once Dad started having strokes, they were confined close to home with Mom as his caregiver. I promised Mom that one day I would take her to Vegas. After we lost Dad, I planned the big trip. Mom started asking when we were going home before we even got to the hotel. She loved to travel but this time she seemed a little frightened. It was so close to Dad's death, I just assumed she was still recovering from that.

FEBRUARY 22, 2013

I am the keynote speaker for the Women Go Red for the American Heart Association. This is the first time Mom will see me as a speaker.

A sweet moment! She's just beaming.

Much resemblance to you, so you will age well too!

Dayna note: I had just moved Mom into a nearby assisted living retirement home and she had never seen me speak at a large public event. We had taken her car away just a few days before because she was beginning to get disoriented on the highway.

I was forever trying to fill her days. She hated being stranded there with all the "old people." She seems a little overwhelmed by the crowd and is having a difficult time following along with any conversations. She herself, always a great conversationalist, never met a stranger. She is not initiating any conversations. She is saying the same things to everyone. Something is not quite right. Glad I have her living near me with some supervision. I make an appointment for her to see her new primary care doctor in the next week.

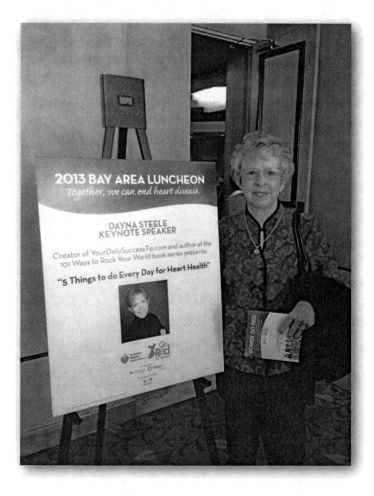

March 20, 2013

My Mom was diagnosed with early stages of Alzheimer's today.

Did she take the test (not sure what it is called)? What was her score? (21)

My Dad has dementia. I visit him everyday after work. I take his dog to visit and his favorite food. The best way to describe it is, that it's a long walk down a hall full of doors to confusing places and I never know which door he has opened or what's coming.

I learned to agree and be positive. Talk about what is going on at the moment.

The decline is excruciating to see.

Dayna note: I took Mom in for a checkup. Doctor asks the simple questions, Mom could not answer most or perform the tasks. Who is the President? Remember three words. Draw a clock. What year is it? Recall these three words. She's laughing. But keeps looking at me for help with the answers. I don't even need to see test results. I know. On this date, we visited with the neurologist for the diagnosis. Just for confirmation. Mom is there and doesn't even acknowledge what the doctor is saying. She just wants to know when we are going to lunch. The doctor tells us that she is well into the stages, maybe halfway already. Smart cookie — she has hidden it well. Now I know what all the notes are for around her apartment. She can't remember. That's why there have been notes for the past six years.

MRI of the brain without contrast

History: 83 year-old with memory loss and dementia.

Multiplanar, multislice MRI of the brain is performed without contrast on a 1.5 Tesla magnet.

Marked hazy increased T2/flair signal is present throughout the pons, suggesting marked chronic small vessel ischemic disease. There is mild chronic small vessel ischemic disease in the white matter of the cerebral hemispheres bilaterally. A moderately large old lacunar infarct is present in the superior right external capsule, extending into the putamen. A few tiny, scattered i old acunar infarcts are present in the basal ganglia bilaterally. No cortical-based infarct is identified. There is no evidence for acute ischemia on diffusion weighted images.

There is no evidence for intracranial mass, mass effect or extra-axial fluid collection. No subacute or chronic blood products are seen.

There is enlargement of the temporal horns, out of proportion to the degree of volume loss than elsewhere with moderate to marked volume loss of the hippocampal formations bilaterally. The appearance suggests Alzheimer's disease. Please correlate clinically. Xanthogranulomatous cysts are incidentally noted within the occipital horns of the lateral ventricles bilaterally.

Normal flow voids are present in the arterial vessels at the skull base and in the dural venous sinuses.

The pituitary, internal auditory canals and visualized cranial nerves at the skull base are unremarkable.

Mild to moderate right mastoid air cell opacification is present. Paranasal sinuses are clear. The patient has undergone previous bilateral cataract surgery.

Impression:

Chronic small vessel ischemic disease is present, mild in the white matter of the cerebral hemispheres and marked in the pons. There are scattered old lacunar infarcts in the basal ganglia bilaterally. No acute intracranial pathology is identified.

There is significant volume loss of the hippocampal formations and enlargement of the temporal horns, out of proportion to the degree of volume loss and ventricular enlargement noted elsewhere in the brain. The appearance is concerning for Alzheimer's disease. Please correlate clinically.

May 6, 2013

Let me tell you a nice story today. My mother, recently diagnosed with Alzheimer's, is absolutely obsessed with astronaut Rick Linnehan. She calls him constantly. He came over for dinner last night and treated her like a date, even posing with her dog. She was giddy. Thank you Rick that will always be a nice memory.

He just became my favorite astronaut as well...KUDOS Rick! What a feel good story, thank you Dayna Steele for sharing that special moment.

Too sweet!! She was telling me all about Rick last week.

Beneath that crusty exterior, beats a heart of gold. He just doesn't like people to know!

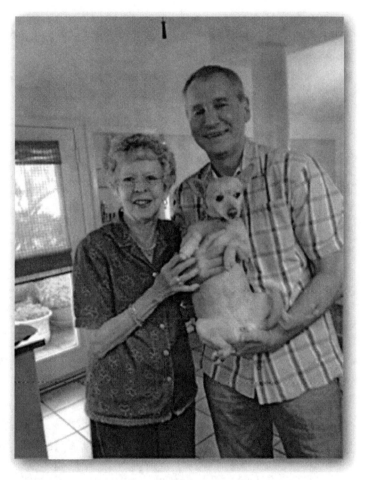

JULY 12, 2013

So if you went to our neighborhood Chick-fil-A today dressed as a cow, you got a free lunch. My mom is in an assisted living facility. The wonderful activities director Bonnie Pate Schoellkopf, made shirts for the residents. A whole bus full of them went. I can't thank this place enough. My Mom is so happy. Alzheimer's Be Damned!

Thanks so much for sharing your Mom with me.

Wonderful story!! The simple things that make magic moments for folks! Thanks for sharing.

PRICELESS!!

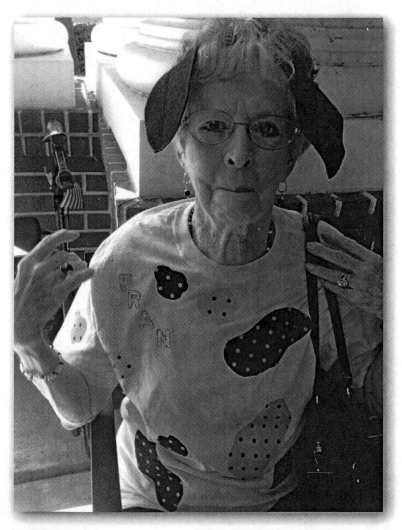

JULY 23, 2013

Posted from Fran's care center activities director Bonnie Pate Schoellkopf: Bingo winner with only eight numbers called.

Go Fran!

Ms. Fran ended up winning 2 more games.

> Dayna note: Mom loved to gamble — lottery cards, bingo, slots — you name it. Bingo was the last activity she could participate in. As confusion set in, other residents and my brother helped her play until we moved from this facility.

SEPTEMBER 8, 2013

Scooter (Dayna's brother) made mom's famous Chicken Spaghetti for her birthday party. Astronaut Rick Linnehan took it on one of his (space) missions. Here he is posing with it tonight next to the package he brought home from space.

Let's try out that package and see if it tastes the same! We will let Rick try first.

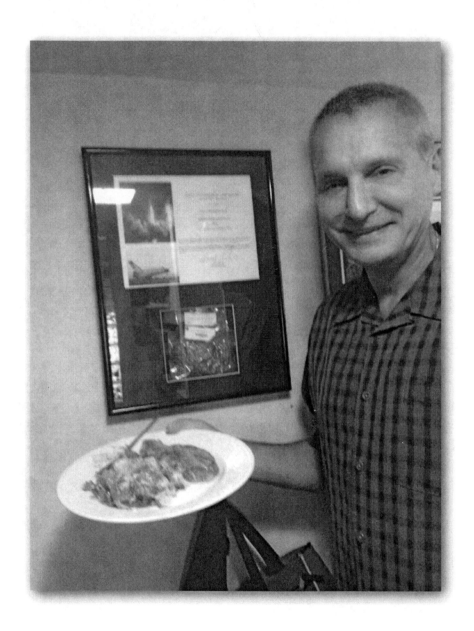

CHICKEN SPAGHETTI (Serves a bunch!)
1 5-6 lb. hen or 2 fryers
    Stew until tender, remove meat from bones, set aside
to cool and then skim fat off broth.
Saute' the following in olive oil:
    2 medium onions, chopped
    1 or 2 cloves garlic, chopped
    3 - 4 ribs celery, cut in small pieces
    2 carrots, cut in small pieces
    1 med. size green pepper, cut in small pieces
Add to chicken broth along with the following:
    1 can cr. of tomato soup
    1 can cr. of mushroom soup
    1 4oz. can mushroom stem & pieces
    1 large can tomatoes (put thru sieve or blender)
    2 small cans tomato sauce
    1 small can chopped black olives
    2 - 3 T. parsley
Season all with:
    salt & pepper to taste
    2-3 T. worcestershire sauce
    2-3 T. chili powder
    2 T. sweet basil
    1 T. sugar
    dash of paprika
Add to chicken pieces:
    1/2 pound velveta cheese (grated)
Cook until tender the following:
    10 - 12 oz. spaghetti

Combine all ingredients and pour into casserole dishes,
covering with grated sharp cheese.
cook for about 45 minutes   - 375º

September 11, 2013

I'm learning:
Mom: I hate those clouds.
Me: Why?
Mom: I don't like them. Make them go away.
Me: OK.
Mom: Thanks. Can we have ice cream?

Me: Sure. Look, I've made some of the clouds go away.
Mom: What are you talking about?
Me: Nothing.

I'm sorry but this is funny. I am like you, look for the positive so you just have to laugh.

When my son and I stopped by her place the other day she told me to come see her apartment, you haven't seen it yet, and even though I had, we acted happy for her to show us again.

Thanks for the honesty and candor that it took to post this, as I know it helps others to see that there is no wrong way, or right way to help someone you love. Just being there is all it takes.

If this is typical of your conversations you are very lucky indeed. In my family, we were not so lucky!

This is the funniest thing I've seen for two days now. Just sent it to my boss. She cracked up too!

September 11, 2013 (Part 2)

Conversation on the way home:
Mom: Why am I in this place?
Me: I have to make sure you are happy and safe because you have a form of dementia.
Mom: (Amazed wide eyed voice) I have DEMENTIA?
Me: Yep.
Mom: (happily onto another subject) Well then ...
Makes me crack up every time. I know. Dark humor ...

Dayna note: It was Mom's 84th birthday — She took her first selfie.

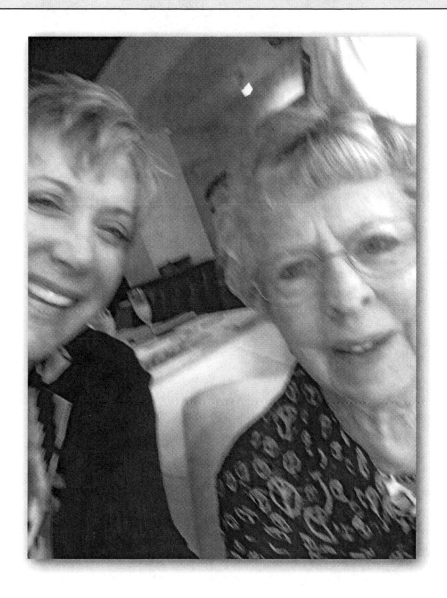

September 25, 2013

Mom has always had a big bowl of Peanut M&M's on a counter or table for as long as I can remember. And she often carried emergency supplies in her purse:

Me: I got you a surprise!

Mom: What is it? (Toddler like anticipation)

Me: The little Halloween packages of Peanut M&M's!

Mom: What's a peanut M&M?

Me: Here try these.

Mom: Oooh these are so good! Can I have more?

Instead of being sad, we look at it this way — we got to see Mom's joy in eating her first Peanut M&M. Again.

The day I learned to reframe was my first day of emotional freedom.

Eating is a very last pleasure in life. When you cannot converse any more, you can share these special moments. Treasure these moments.

September 30, 2013

Me: Mom do you remember your neighbors in Quail Valley?

Mom: Ummmm, Raynell and that other woman.

Me: Pearlie?

Mom: Yes, Raynell and Pearlie. I can't remember any others.

Me: What about when you lived in Country Place?

Mom: That Keffenberger woman.

Me: You mean Betty you played bingo with?

Mom: Yes, that's the only name I remember. And those other people were there too.

Me: Do you remember the most you have won on a bingo lottery card:

Mom: Oh yes. That was a few weeks ago, I won $100. I've also won $50 and $30 in the last couple of years. And of course, there is the time I won $300 on that nickel machine at Delta Downs as I was walking out the door. You know I win at bingo almost every day now right?

Me: You go girl!

Off to the corner store to buy more bingo lottery cards ...

Clever and touching!

These little nuggets are awesome!

Dayna note: Thanks all. I have to find the humor or the sadness and the anger will take over. My patience was horribly short today but she just called to tell me she won at bingo three times and won the final winner take all pot. Happy as a clam. Is it too early for wine?

October 14, 2013

Mom: I didn't know your middle name was Frances.

Me: Yep. Named after you.

Mom: Are you sure about that?

Me: Fairly.

(Mom's name is Frances.)

I once walked in on my grandmother watching the Playboy channel.
When she saw I was standing there she said "they've never done this
on Young and the Restless before." I had to leave the room for a few
minutes then calmly came back and changed the channel to Y&R. As

difficult as the disease is, try and remember the funny and touching moments.

October 20, 2013

Mom has brain bleed, not so-nice side effect sometimes from Alzheimer's or so I've learned. It is like a stroke. She is having a hard time obeying commands, trouble putting words together, and her fidgeting has increased 10 times. So much so, they had to put what looked like giant white boxing gloves on her hands and restrain her. The only coherent things she said yesterday were 'do you know who my daughter is' and in regards to the gloves, 'I am NOT paying for these things.' Had to smile …

Never get sick on a weekend. Even the greatest med center in the world has non-existent infrastructure on the weekends. Nothing is open, no valet, and the only café in the hospital is nasty. Apparently no one really cares much on the weekends. I hear this is typical throughout the Houston system. It most definitely is at Memorial Hermann. Too bad!! We really could be world class with a touch of more effort.

Singing songs from your Mom's era is very calming. Songs are the first thing we learn as a child and the last things we forget, as we get older.

Be strong and do your best to be a good advocate for her. Make peace with the fact that some things are simply not within your control.

October 22, 2013

Mom has been promoted from ICU to the Stroke Rehab floor. A big positive move so soon after her little 'event.' Her nurse James is a rocker. I love him. Mom has proven to be Houdini reincarnated. Wrist and body restraints ain't got nothing on this feisty one! One more thing … I now know where my truck-driver snore came from.

Sending you love fellow sandwich generation person! Takes a village.

Great news! Tell Fran to give those therapists H, E, double L.

OCTOBER 23, 2013

It has been a challenging few days. Mom had a stroke sometime late last week and I discovered it when I picked her up Saturday morning. We are the lucky ones. She was just released to rehab and we are waiting on the ambulance to transport her now. I don't know what we would have done these past couple of days (though it seemed like years) without her nurse James. Memorial Herman should know that he is one of their hidden gems. (He was later awarded for his commitment) Just bought Mom a brush from the gift shop. She has informed me that she is not leaving until her hair is done…

At least she has her priorities straight!

Gotta love those Southern women!

Dayna note: James was given the weekly Standing Ovation Award by this hospital not long after I wrote this. Nurses could learn from him. Great compassion and communication. That's all we ask for. If I had to do it all over again, I would not have let them do as many procedures as they did, not as much medicine. Many will argue with me but why prolong the inevitable? I would only keep her out of pain.

OCTOBER 26, 2013

Sons Dack and Nick have locked me out of the house. Brother Scooter, Aunt and Uncle, have taken over care. Friends Sid and Cathy have reserved the sky suite in the Quarter. Wonder Husband Charles has kidnapped me and we are in the plane on our way to New Orleans. Nervous to leave her but this caregiver is about to give out.

Caregivers make better caregivers when they take care of themselves too!

As much traveling as you do, you should know "Oxygen mask on you first, then you can help others!" Hugs.

You have to relax — re-charge ... after all who will take care of everyone if you get sick??

OCTOBER 27, 2013

First full coherent sentence since stroke:
Mom: My hair looks like shit.
Me: (laughing) Yes it does!
Then my amazing stylist arrives and gives her a do! We wheelchair her around the whole damn place to show it off. Thanks Lisa Lingo.
Me: Mimi can you smile for me?
Mom: No, I don't feel like smiling.
Me: I take a picture of her frowning and show it to her.
Mom: I don't like that picture. *Laughs*

A woman who doesn't feel like smiling, and doesn't, despite pressure to do so, is a woman after my own heart. Plus she's beautiful, regardless!! (Hug).

She looks so much like you.

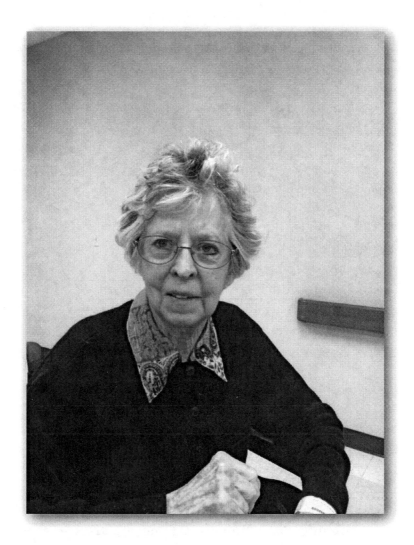

NOVEMBER 1, 2013

Several months ago, the phone calls from Mom started to increase substantially. Then two weeks ago they stopped abruptly. Yesterday Mom learned to use her phone again, calling me every few minutes. Never been so happy to hear that ring. Not sure it will ever drive me crazy again.

My mother used to tell me there was something wrong with her phone. Found out she was trying to ring me up with her TV remote.

My mom had Alzheimer's, and passed away almost 6 years ago. I'd love for my phone to ring and her voice would be on the other end.

What a precious post. I will be thankful for calls from my parents and will not take them for granted.

NOVEMBER 3, 2013

Mom adores astronaut Rick Linnehan. He surprised her with a visit today. They are out for a stroll while I watch and smile. Rick is one of the good guys. He knows how she feels about him. He asked if he could come and see her. Very Special!

True definition of PRICELESS!

I bet Rick doesn't care if she recognizes him … the most selfless don't … it's not about us it is time with them (your Mom)

Dayna note: She couldn't remember his name but did grin when she saw him through the window walking up. It is so important for friends and family to visit no matter what stage of Alzheimer's the patient is experiencing. Even if the patient doesn't recognize you, the visit still means the world to them. The patient will always need to know someone still cares about them.

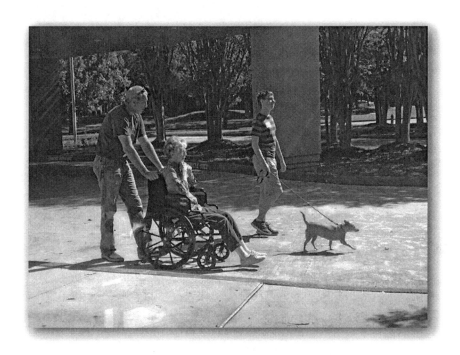

November 5, 2013

People more often than not don't die of Alzheimer's. They die from poor judgment or the lack of any judgment. Mom's doctor in rehab thinks her stroke was caused by malnutrition and dehydration. She had gotten into the habit of drinking Cokes all day — which curbed her appetite and kept her from drinking water. She returned to her apartment yesterday and is not happy with the contents of her refrigerator — water, Boost protein drink and Diet Dr Pepper (and wine). Yes, she was happy with the wine. I did not fall far from the tree…

> *Going through something similar with Mom (although not nearly as severe). Dehydration caused some major problems. Water was never her forte, either! Sending*
> *Empathy vibes …*

*I snuck wine into mom when she was in the Alzheimer's care faculty...
She kept two of her nice wine glasses there, one for me and one for her.
The facility frowned upon it because of potential drug interference. Uh,
come on, really ... I told them to stick it ... and they turned a blind eye*

*In his last weeks my dad asked for whiskey — and he almost never drank.
We got a tiny bottle of Crown Royal Maple and put just a drop on his
tongue and he moaned in appreciation - that was the last response we got
from him, and he died 36 hours later.*

NOVEMBER 7, 2013

One of the hardest things about this whole process is learning to let go
and let other people take care of me. I'm used to doing that for others
and am very uncomfortable on the receiving end. Gwen Griffin, Cathy
Arroyo, Cheryl Evans, Charles Justiz, and Dack Justiz are just a few of
the people who are holding me up right now. That and my cousin Kay
Jenkins, who owns Doc's Boutique-Retail Therapy at It's Best, brought
me bubble bath, a soothing candle, a bottle of wine and two glasses that
hold entire bottles of wine.

You deserve a bubble bath, a big a@$ glass of wine and some time to yourself!!!

NOVEMBER 9, 2013

Even when you're losing your mind, a pedicure can always make a girl happy.

What a smile!

Looks like she is happy!

She's not losing her mind...her memory is locked up and she forgot where she put the key.

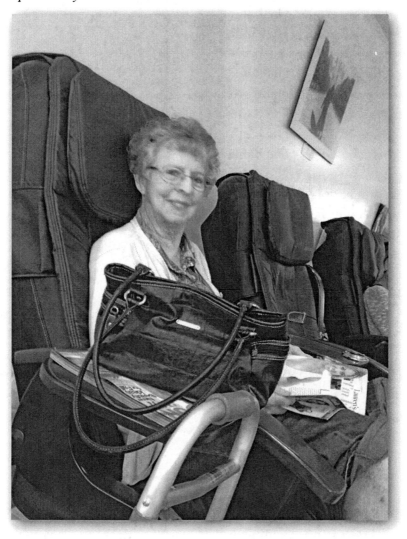

NOVEMBER 12, 2013

Where are we going? The bank.
Where are we going? The bank.
Where are we going? The bank.
Where are we going? The bank.
Where are we going? The bank.
Where are we going? The bank.
Where are we going? The bank.
Where are we going? The bank.
Where are we going? The bank.
Where are we going? The bank.
Where are we going? The bank.
I figured it out. It is Karma for all the times I said, "Are we there yet?"

Sad but Funny!

Way to find the silver lining...And find the humor.

As my dear mother always said, " you're gonna pay for your raisin' ..."

I do have a little window into your situation ... our mentally challenged daughter does the same thing! It can be maddening, but keeping your good humor is a ready defense against moments of despair.

NOVEMBER 15, 2013

We are 7 ½ months into official Alzheimer's (diagnosed 3-20-2013). Well, I knew it was coming but it wasn't a dramatic, teary thing. I thought it would be when it did come. In fact, it was a pretty straight-forward, matter-of-fact question from Mom. She simply asked the question and then followed it with a chuckle and a "Sorry, I'm getting older" comment. I replied, "That's ok, we are ALL getting older every day." Her question? … "What's your name?"

Hugs for you!! At least she has a sense of humor.

It's heartbreaking for you. It's heartbreaking for her and terrifying at the same time.

Your Mom hasn't really forgotten who you are, she has just forgotten how to remember your name. The heartwarming part is that despite the difficulties she has her daughter by her side. She is a lucky Mom.

November 20, 2013

She may not remember my name but she does remember her dog's name. Sandy. Never underestimate the power of love for an animal.

But she certainly still understands your love, Dayna.

Dayna note: Taking away her dog was harder than taking away her car. The dog was starting to be too much, tripping others, getting loose, wrapping around walkers. For her safety and safety of others, had to be done.

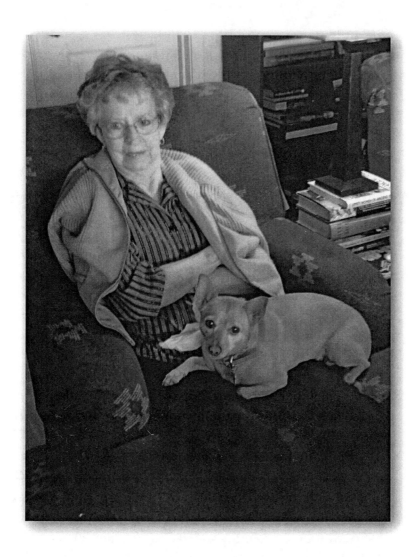

December 1, 2013

Mom: These are pretty. Where did they come from?
Me: You made them.
Mom: I made them?

Me: Yes, you used to make hundreds of these for friends and family as well as for our tree.

Mom: I did?

Me: Yes, really, you made these.

Mom: (picks one up, really examines it close for a minute or so)

Mom: Wow! I was REALLY good!!

Me: Yes, you were.

Dayna, your mother taught me how to make these. We made the exact one in this photo with the triangles. I think my mom still has it. She also taught me how to tie my shoes ... Love her!

My grandmother made some like these too. They are keepsakes. I cherish putting them on the tree every year.

OMG ... I have a container full of these!!!

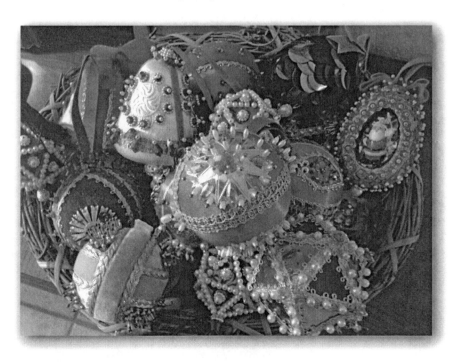

December 4, 2013

Mom is now calling 15 to 20 times per day and leaving a message. Former roommate and astronaut Edward Lu asked me what she says in these messages.
They are usually short, like this:
Getting my hair done.
Where are you?
I'm eating lunch
I don't know where you are?
Not sure why I called.
Taking a walk.
Eating dinner.
Watching "Wheel of Fortune."
Ed says. " Oh you mean like a Twitter feed."
I laughed out loud. Exactly. Just like Twitter feed.

Sorry to hear! Thinking of you. Facebook needs that button instead of Like.

At least your mom can dial the phone. I had to take mom's away when she called the operator each time she phoned me. I didn't discover this until the bill came in $450. Amazingly they were sympathetic and waved the charges.

So beautiful you can find the humor amongst your family's rougher parts of the journey.

The thing about your posts is you are saying and experiencing the exact thing that so many are in dealing with the disease. You have an uncanny way of making it real and new. Thanks for sharing. I certainly feel your pain.

December 7, 2013

Mom decided we needed to have a jewelry show. So we are having a jewelry show. With wine! Now. If you are in my area drop by our house. She'll last till about 5:00 p.m. These are pearls she designed and strung a while ago. Her pre-Alzheimer's career. No guarantees on how long the wine will last …

Oh if I was in the area I'd SO be there. And I'd bring some wine just to be on the safe side!

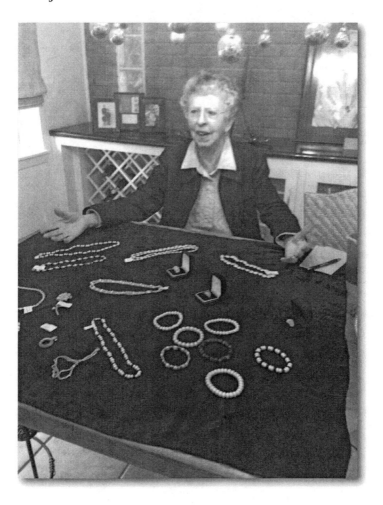

DECEMBER 13, 2013

A simple explanation of this horrific disease: You go from beginning to infant to toddler to teenager to adult. When the "long goodbye" starts, you go from adult to teenager to toddler to infant to end. We figure Mom's journey started about five years ago but she hid it so damn well. We are entering toddler stage now with the terrible 2's rearing their ugly head …
Eat your green beans.
No!
Wear your shoe inserts.
No!
Drink your water.
No!
Eat all your dinner.
No!
Put your seat belt on.
No!
Stay right there.
(wanders off)
Do you want candy?
Yes!
This is one constant in all of our lives. ALL of us always want candy!!

> *When my mom was in the childhood stage of this disease we had the seatbelt talk … she finally said ok but couldn't find it. My daughter, in the back seat, handed it to mom, who giggled and innocently said, "Well there it is … I guess it's always better from the back".… and then amazingly … realized how that sounded and turned red … still makes me laugh.*

> *My wife hadn't spoken a word except, "Yay," for months. One day I gave her a bag of M&M Peanuts … she grabbed them … began to devour and said, "I just love these." I almost fainted!*

December 17, 2013

In a moment of lucidity, Mom told me there is plenty to do at her assisted living home and plenty of people to talk to "though they are old." What she added took my breath away.

Mom: I just get so depressed here. I don't have a family.

Me: But Mom you do. I am your family. Charlie, the boys and I are here all the time.

Mom: Yes, but I don't have a family or home to take care of. I don't have anything to care for. I can't drive. I can't cook, there's no house, there's no yard for me to take care of. I can't even have my Sandy anymore (her dog who kept pulling her down and tripping others).

That made it so clear to me. This woman who made me who I am — the person who loves to take care of my husband, my boys, my family, my home, my friends, etc. She is a nurturer and that is who taught me. So, the question is — what do I get her to take care of?

There's a story about Ronald Reagan that I love. He loved to rake the leaves from the reflecting pond at his ranch. It was something simple that he really enjoyed. So every morning a Secret Service agent had the task of throwing leaves into the pool. Something simple that gave him purpose.

December 31, 2013

2013 has been a year of challenges and lessons. We toast another year with Mom. Thanks for being a part of our journey. I could not do this without all of you. P.S. What is that? Champagne. Why? It's New Years Eve. Why? It's what you drink on this night. Ok (drinks). Yuck! I don't like this. Oh, I do … here I'll take that. Happy New Year Y'all!

I had many conversations with my Mom; dementia and Alzheimer's can take a toll on your nerves, but not your sense of humor Dayna. Keep your head high, remember the great times and remember that it is a disease despite it seeming like a full blown attack or test on your self control. It WILL be ok, hang in there, you are doing great!

One in nine people age 65 and older (11 percent) has Alzheimer's disease.
                    - Alzheimer's Association 2015 Overview Report

2 0 1 4 :

WHERE ARE WE GOING?

JANUARY 3, 2014

We stopped at Nazar's Fine Jewelry. Mom strung pearls for Nazar's for 27 years. A whirlwind tour for her today!

> *I just remembered that your mom re-strung my mom's pearls (my dad brought them back from Japan in 1965). I also have a beautiful bracelet she designed with both my boys' names on it! Your mom is precious and always has been.*

> **Dayna note: Mom did not know who they were. Last visit to Nazar's.**

JANUARY 26, 2014

Haven't had one of these for you in awhile. She's getting a little worse, more like a demanding toddler you cannot reason with. With that said, we still look for smiles where we can find them.

Mom: (snickering) Looks like someone tried to make you a bracelet and it is way to small.

Me: That's a napkin ring.

Mom: What's a napkin ring?

Me: You pull the napkin through it to make the table look nice when you set the places.

Mom: Well that's silly.

Me: That's what I've always thought too …

> *Reed and I send Jason to work every day with a piece of blue painter's tape around his napkin. We be all fancy.*

> *Love that you are sharing it … and, she is definitely right about napkin rings.*

January 27, 2014

She's got a bad cough and we are at the doctor's office. I'm on a business call and she keeps trying to show me something. I finally look over. Well damn. That's me (in a magazine). Mom is tickled as we say in Texas ...

She shared the article. She is so proud.

That's so sweet that she recognized you in the magazine! I'm glad she still has reasons to smile. Rode w/ her in the elevator this afternoon and we were talking tennis and how much she used to play.

Made me tear up. These moments are gold! Memories for the future, and also bittersweet.

February 2, 2014

She loves Texas Lottery Bingo cards. When I travel, I send a few in a card, every day or so. Keeps her from getting quite as frantic when I leave town. It is the little things ...

I called bingo for her group on Friday. She didn't win anything this time, so hopefully the cards bring her better luck.

I hope she wins!

I remember when you were leaving the air to move to California. You were doing well until your Mom showed up in the studio and you just couldn't hold back your emotions about leaving us! It's your turn now to be there for her and you are doing very well!

FEBRUARY 11, 2014

Is it too early for wine?

> *I heard a DJ this morning on Saturday radio say, " If you are going to drink all day, you have to start in the morning," so drink up!*

> *It's 5 o'clock somewhere!*

> *I have heard after 11 am ... unless you did not sleep the night before ... then you can drink anytime you damn well please.*

> *For you or Aunt Fran? Either way, it is never too early!*

FEBRUARY 14, 2014

Mom is getting more and more frantic when she comes over. She cannot sit still for more than a couple of minutes. She goes back-and-forth between the library, the kitchen and the bathroom. I kept hearing the most awful loud noise coming from the kitchen so I went to investigate. Every time she leaves the kitchen she puts the bar stools back where they go. It's getting harder for her to figure out how to do that but she still insists on putting them back each and every time, properly. Dear people — who-have-a-penis-in-my-house and never put the bar stools back — I come by it honestly.

> *My Mom has been nervously straightening and moving things to the point that no one can find things. Daily treasure hunt!*

> *It's never easy dealing with this type of thing. At least you can find the humor in it. I guess if we don't laugh we will cry.*

Alzheimer's a terrible malady. I was the caregiver for my father-in-law for the last year of his life. The last 4 months were a humbling experience. The hardest job I have ever had. You learn patience you never thought you had, tolerance for things that always aggravated you, and a greater appreciation for the person who used to be.

February 24, 2014

It seems like ages that I told you how happy I was Mom could use a phone and call me again after her stroke. I was warned by her care facility that this would eventually start. And it has. Call after call, voicemail after voicemail, within minutes if not seconds of each one. I know I will miss her, her calls, and the sound of her voice when she is gone but this does take its toll. I'm having a hard time finding something humorous to say about this. So, the pressure is on, make me laugh:

My father-law did something similar except he would call 911 to invite them to lunch.

My father had Alzheimer's and had one of those emergency buttons around his neck. For some reason his widow took it from him and hid it. One of the times she left him alone, he found the button and pressed it a few times. Ambulance showed up, and the widow got a phone call. She hauled ass home from whatever she was doing to find dad happy as a clam with a captive audience, and one of the emergency fellows even served him his coffee. This memory of my father makes me smile to this day.

I will send you my mother's number and she can call her!

MARCH 7, 2014

Mom: Where are we going?
Me: To get a pedicure.
Mom: Where are we going?
Me: To get a pedicure.
Mom: Where are we going?
Me: To get a pedicure.
Mom: Where are we going?
Me: To get a pedicure.
Mom: Where are we going?
Me: To get a pedicure.
Mom: Where are we going?
Me: To get a pedicure.
(Few seconds of silence)
Mom: I really need a pedicure, think we could get one soon?
Mom: Yes! (Thrilled) You are really sweet. Thanks.

I had a dearly beloved patient for all of 28 years of my practice. The few years she rapidly progressed through Alzheimer's to that despairingly HORRIBLE place where she did not recognize me (and I took care of her mother and grown daughters, too). Her daughter brought her in for a full check up including a Pap smear. Midway through all our favorite exams she startled me by sitting bolt upright exclaiming, "You're Dr. Halpern! Aren't you?" Amazing when that brain synapse sparks or what might cause it! I laughed then and saved my tears for later. But anything I can do to help you (including designated driver happy hour) I am here. Keep writing.

I have had the same conversation with my mom who also has Alzheimer's. You just have to see the humor!

March 19, 2014

Mom brought Charlie a picture of her and 'his mom.' It is actually a picture of Snowlily Lu, astronaut Edward Lu's mom. If she has to get moms confused, Snowlily is a great one to do it with. Thanks for sharing your mom with us Ed!

I just thought of her yesterday when I wore some of her pearls that I bought from her. Lovely.

March 24, 2014

Mom brings over pictures that excite her. This one is when astronaut Tom Henricks brought the Olympic torch home. Is there any question who I look like?

You were photo bombing before it was cool!!!

You are a Mini-me. I remember that flight. I was the STS-78 crew secretary.

I love that she is selecting certain photos with handsome astronauts.

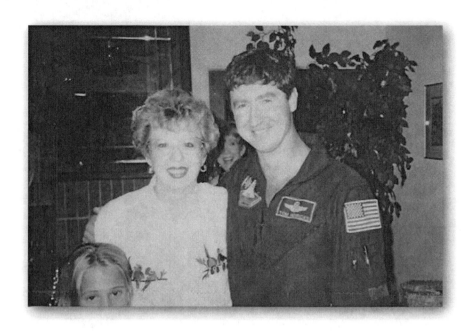

March 27, 2014

Mom: Why are all these people sending me paperwork?
Me: That's my friend and those are note cards. I asked if they would send you notes while I was on vacation. Guess you are still getting some.
Mom: Who lives in Vermont? It's snowing there.
Me: That would be my friend AmyBeth
Mom: Who is Liesbeth? She sure writes a lot. Is she really crazy as she says?
Me: Yes.
Mom: Who is Chris Nocera? He sent a lot of lottery bingo cards.
Me: He's a local TV producer.
Mom: Do you know him?
Me: Yes. He is a good friend.
Mom: Tell him only one card was a winner and I want more.
Me: Yes Mom.

She must have misunderstood. You are the crazy one.

I find it both amazing and heartwarming how you can frame a sad situation with such good humor. Hang in there; we're rooting for you.

> Dayna note: Thanks for your wonderful kind words. Please know that this is how I am coping with everything. There are days when I drop her off and cry all the way home. I have to find humor so that I can keep going for her.

. 2014

Your mom is enjoying the game — with Bonnie Schoellkopf.

You sure look like your mom, God bless her!

I love that you have beauty shop day together.

> Dayna note: This seemingly mild post really upset me this day. Mom hated baseball ...

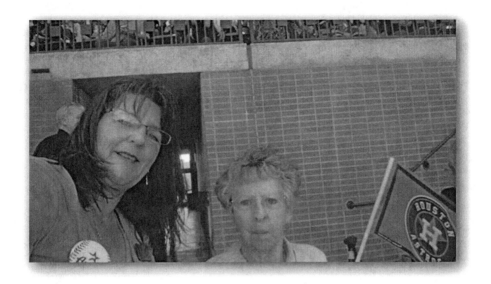

April 15, 2014

Wonderful friend Michelle Moog-Koussa and her amazing son Gregory joined us for a few days. Michelle and Gregory were like new company every day for Mom. And so sweet, to just keep re-introducing themselves! Like in the movie Groundhog Day ...

Love, Love!!

So much love. So cute you all are!

April 23, 2014

One of the hardest things for me has been learning not to argue or correct her.

When she says she played tennis where her townhouse was, I say, "Yep and you were great." She played tennis in Quail Valley not in Country Place.

When she says she played tennis until last week, I say, "Yep, and you were great." She last played tennis 20 years ago or more.

When she says she will play tennis in a few weeks when her foot feels better, I say, "Yep, and you will be great." And she will be.

Yoga breath. Ommmmmmmmmmmmm!!!

Great form!!

Those tennis ladies lived and breathed tennis. What a life! So happy she remembers that good time in her life.

I went to a garage sale in Quail Valley and purchased some books that had your name in them. I asked the lady having the sale if she knew you and she said, "I should, she's my baby girl."

April 26, 2014

She taught me how to cook, hands down my favorite hobby. Now I return the favor …

My Mom just quoted your mom the other day on "how to make a proper roux."

Looks like fun to me! Enjoy your time together.

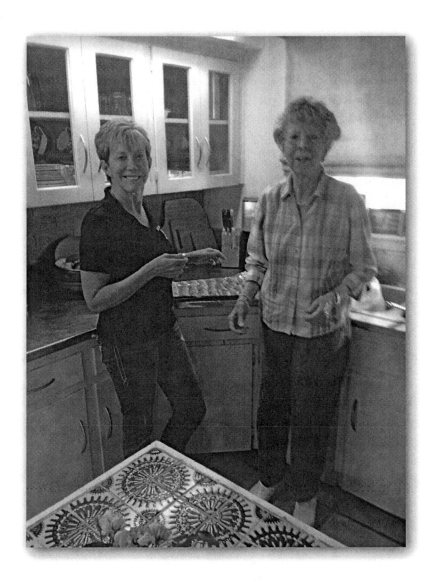

APRIL 27, 2014

I had a puzzle made out of one of Mom's tennis pictures. Enlisted Cheryl Evans and Aunt Mary. I'm drinking wine. And watching.

Great idea. Where did you have the puzzle made?

Shutterfly.com!

Is my mother getting tipsy with you again?

What a great idea! Putting the pieces together…WOW!!

APRIL 28, 2014

Mom loves Girl Scout Cookies. Even more so, she likes to sneak them out of my pantry. This cookie caper gives her great joy. We are running low on Thanks-A-Lots, her favorite.
If you are one of those amazing parents who got stuck with cookies this year, I'll buy 'em. I'll buy all of 'em. Stat!

I think I know a guy who has at least one extra box he can spare.

There is a guide on how to pair wine with Girl Scout cookies.

APRIL 30, 2014

Before we knew what was going on, I would occasionally check Mom's bank accounts to make sure she had money, no problems, etc. There was cash disappearing every week — she always laughed it off and made an excuse. Turns out she was spending a couple of hundred dollars every month on the Texas Lottery Lucky Gems Bingo cards. I explained over and over again that she didn't really have the income to do that. Now, I let it go — it is one of the less than a handful of things she cares about anymore. Each card is good for about 45 minutes entertainment and she gets really sad if she runs out of cards. This is her obsession … along with pilfering my Girl Scout cookies.

If you find these anywhere in the state of Texas, buy all you can afford and I will pay you back and cover postage. These have to last as long as her mind does …

Can I ask why it has to be this particular bingo?

I imagine that you could use something like black poster paint to recycle the cards she's scratched off. Might save you some time and money.

I know from experience that Alzheimer's patients can't learn new things. They simply can't. Repainting used cards sounds like an ideal solution. Good luck! I know how important this is to you and your mom …

> Dayna note: Tried everything — has to be these — disease too far progressed to teach her new things. She just doesn't get it. Thanks all! Go hunt! Tried the iPad. That was interesting.

May 2, 2014

Sometimes 'family' is not necessarily a blood relative. One of mom's dearest longtime friends stopped by for a night during a road trip earlier this week. Mom wasn't sure who she was, but true to form (and the way I was raised), was extremely nice and pretended to know her. Mom and Tess traveled many, many times together. Mom remembers the trips but not the company. It was heartwarming for me and heartbreaking for Tess. So, we drank wine. A lot of wine. And we cried. A lot of tears. I needed this family visit more than you'll ever know Tess …

They need a button bigger than "Like" for stories that hit you right in the heart.

Tess Tancred Nelson: You said it so well, Dayna, it was a wonderful visit for me too with Fran and you. Nice picture — she looks just like Fran on the outside — I have a new different friend now. She took off her bracelet and gave it to me. I have many pieces of gold jewelry that I bought from her through 40 years, but I will cherish this one — makes me sad and happy! Your mom has always been proud to have you as her daughter and you deserve it now more than ever.

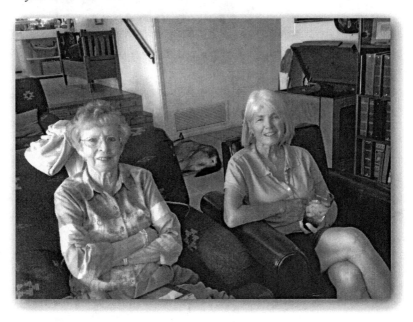

MAY 09, 2014

Her nickname is Flo. My mother is gone, well most of the time. It has been that way for a while now and getting worse. My mother has Alzheimer's. The woman I knew as Mommy now relies on me for everything. That's okay. She taught me to love, to cook, to do for others, to only spend what you have, to write handwritten thank you notes, to play tennis (well, she tried on that one). She let me leave for college when I was 16, she told me about sex without ever batting an eye or cringing, she told me it was best in love. She rejoiced in my pregnancies and she babysat even when she didn't want to. I think she has a big crush on Charlie the Wonder Husband. I miss my mom. Stop working. Go call your mom. Even better, spend the weekend with her. Business and success will wait for you on this one. Happy Mother's Day to you and yours.

These posts are both heartwarming and heartbreaking. Thank you so much for sharing!

Sometimes the person who has been there for everyone else needs someone to be there for them.

May 13, 2014

Mom was just over for dinner. My aunt and uncle were over as well. After they all left, it hit me. I can't hear her old voice. It is so overwhelming; I can't remember what she was like before this. Sad. Very sad.

I remember when I first noticed my mom had lost her executive function. She had no idea how to change clothes into her nightgown, she couldn't break down the task into its component parts. It is the only time I cried during her decline. It is an insidious disease. You know I love you! You are a great daughter. Your mom would be proud of you how you have cared for her.

All of us who have walked that path remember that moment ... that realization that they are gone far before they are gone. Just remember, you are not alone. We mourn with you. Be not afraid.

Look for old recordings, movies, and even voice mails. I still have some of my mother's last voice mails on my cell. What a treasure.

May 24, 2014

Mom was well known for the quality of work she did stringing high-end pearls and designing jewelry for individuals. She remembers she did it but does not know how anymore. So, my youngest son and I taught ourselves how to make stretch bracelets for her. She always wears one and will sell one off her wrist for $5 for bingo money. She said to me earlier this week, " When are you going to make some more of those bracelets I make?"

I always suspected there were multiple Dayna's – that you had yourself cloned at A&M so you could accomplish more.

There are certain events in life that transform your life into "before the event and after the event." The event that changed my life also changed me into a different person. I will never be the person I was before. It's simply not possible. Hugs.

Please understand if I say nothing, it doesn't mean I've not been touched by your updates. It just means that sometimes they leave me speechless.

May 31, 2014

Change is not a good thing for a memory patient but sometimes it is necessary. We have moved mom from an upstairs unit into a smaller, downstairs unit. Worst thing? Cable change has not gone smoothly.

Called last Tuesday:

On hold for 30 minutes.

Gave up.

Went online.

Said click on Mover's Edge.

Not an active link.

Finally found Mover's Edge.

Filled out all.

It then says 'call this #.'

WTF?

Called the number.

No one answered.

She's having a meltdown over the TV today.

Call Comcast.

Finally get tech services.

Explain all.

He says, what is Mover's Edge?'

Oh for God's sakes — it's part of your company.

Finally gets me to a 'moving specialist.'

Moving specialist "that will be $6."

Me: No it won't.

He agrees, says all is done, so sorry, now transferring you to an activation rep.

What?

Transfers me to a number that starts the process all over.

1 click #1 for tech help.

I get a recording: 'that number is no longer in service.'

I tweet a nasty gram to Comcast.

Write this.

Going home to drink wine.

The End.

Love, Dayna.

Wine makes everything Better.

I think I threatened to throw my stuff in the lake — then I realized they would just charge me for another one!

That's why I got Netflix.

Enjoy your wine.

> Dayna note: Comcast did finally contact me after this post went a little viral. All done now. Probably scared some guy name Joe in tech services. Crazy-ass woman on the phone. Until we find a cure and a cause, Alzheimer's is going to increase which means more and more families will go through this. Large companies need to adjust their policies as well as train their people for these situations. It is hard enough without this sort of customer service.

JUNE 11, 2014

When I was a teen, Mom was an avid tennis player in Quail Valley. She even went to work for Tennis great John Newcombe at Newk's Racquet Club when it opened in the subdivision. She continued to play long after I left the house. She probably hasn't touched a racquet for more than 20 years. With Alzheimer's, she thinks she played until a few weeks ago and is disappointed they don't have courts at Regal Estates. Keeps saying if they did, she'd be out there playing. So here comes neighbor Cheryl Evans — once again coming up with something spectacular for one of us. Here is the door decoration she surprised Mom with yesterday.

That's too precious. Such a thoughtful gesture!

That was so kind.

Dayna note: She lived at the end of La Costa by the golf course. They sold the house to basketball great Rick Barry and family when he joined the Rockets. Mom once told him he really should consider playing basketball for a living. She only read the tennis section in the sports pages.

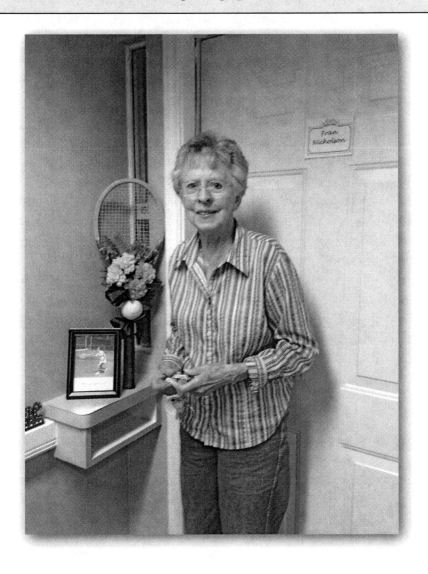

JUNE 16, 2014

Getting into a rough patch here. She calls up to 30 times a day because she doesn't remember calling. She'll ask 15 times where are we going, one after the other. She wants her dog back even though we did that last week and she called four hours later demanding we pick the dog up. There are so many hard parts to this journey. The hardest, of course, is losing your mom. Even though it looks like her, it isn't her anymore. Another hard part is dropping 'remember' and 'I told you' from your vocabulary. Oh, and she called me ' hey lady' today. I swear I started laughing because all I could hear was Jerry Lewis ...

> *The 'remember' part is the hardest for me so far. I want so much to help her to do so. I feel like if I give her enough to jog her memory, she will remember. Sometimes it works, but rarely. Love you and so sorry we're on this journey together, but thankful to have your wisdom and humor.*

> *Bless you for laughing instead of crying.*

> *You have to laugh to keep from crying. Once she put her girdle on top of her pants and we fell on the bed laughing so hard as we were trying to get that darn thing off. Who wears girdles any more these days?*

JUNE 22, 2014

We are gone on a 30-day family flying adventure. Mom was very concerned about me being gone for that long. I finally got her to voice her biggest fear: "Well, who is going to get me into foolishness while you are gone?"

> *Aunt Mary of course!*

She's lucky she will miss you.

Sounds like she was in her right mind.

JULY 12, 2014

Mom took a minor fall yesterday. At this point in the disease with her age she is frailer each and every day. Seems to be okay — just bruised and a little sore. All at Regal Estates keeping an eye on her and I appreciate all they do. So, what happened? The amazing and fabulous Bonnie Schoellkopf took a group of her seniors to Chick-fil-A dressed as cows to you get a free lunch (her second year to do this). She had cow shirts for all of them. One lost her balance, grabbed another's shoulder and they all went down like dominoes. Of course, the first thing I thought was ... cow tipping.

OMG! Your crack me up. Cow tipping!

Humor goes a long way dealing with Alzheimer's. So glad Ms. Fran is ok.

OH Moo....

LMBO.

JULY 23, 2014

One of the Apollo astronauts I talk to occasionally hangs up when he is through talking to me, rarely saying goodbye. I used to think I had offended him. Now I just know it is coming and that is the way he is. He doesn't have time for small talk. Now Mom does it ...
Me: Hello!

Mom: Where are you?

Me: In a meeting (or out of town or in my office or somewhere).

Mom: When are you coming to get me?

Me: No, I'm in a meeting (or out of town or in my office or somewhere).

Mom: So you're not coming to get me?

Me: No, I'm in a meeting (or out of town or in my office or somewhere) but I'll be there (fill in the blank).

Mom: Oh. (Click)

I now think of her as an astronaut. Or maybe an alien? Soon there will be a goodbye and I won't like that one. So I can do without goodbyes for now.

All my friends in Iowa do that. Is it an Iowa thing?

That's what they do in the movies! No one ever says "Goodbye" in the movies! They just hang up! Therefore, it's obvious; your mom is a MOVIE STAR!!

Maybe your Apollo astronaut friend doesn't like goodbye's either …

August 2, 2014

Just when you think you have your emotions in check, the smallest thing can set you off. Or a chain of small things … Today is the third day of Daynamus — a family joke that started years ago and stays around — the twelve days of my birthday because I always found a way to celebrate for as long as possible. Yesterday, I was looking for a recipe and came across Mom's Lemon Jell-O Cake. She had a whole box of my favorites to send me off to my first apartment. Mom has made this for me every year for my birthday until last year. This second year knowing I would once again do without my favorite birthday cake had me feeling a little melancholy yesterday. She was over for dinner last night; Charlie bought a coffee mug and card for her to give me as a Daynamus surprise last night. She used to say this to me as a kid and started repeating it over and over the last year. She seems to have forgotten the saying as recently as a few weeks ago. I opened the gift and lost it … still a little weepy this morning over it but know it will mean the world to me till the day I die. So, as you follow along and support me on this journey, I say to you, "How much do I love you? A bushel and a peck and a hug around the neck."

You brought a smile and a happy tear with this. My grandmother also said that to me so many years ago. Thanks for the reminder, and to your Mom who continues to touch so many lives even though she may not appreciate it.

My mom still sings this to my grandchildren and to my young nieces and nephews. Perfect song for making one feel loved and Cherished!

I love reading your updates.

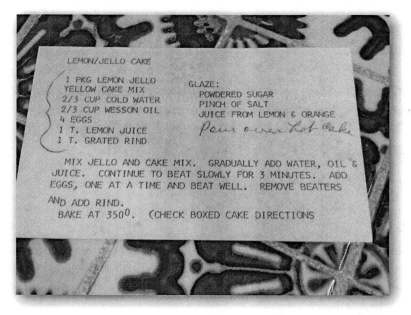

AUGUST 13, 2014

My rock star neurologist brother-in-law tried to explain to me what was next a few months ago — that Dayna her daughter that she calls and talks about is completely different from Dayna her daughter who comes to visit and takes care of her and calls her back. Confused? Yep. That's how this crazy disease works. So things go like this: Mom: Calls me 32 times, one after the other. She leaves me short snippets of messages that mainly consist of are you coming to see me or get me? Me: Finally calling back, " Mom I see you called several times. What's up? "Mom: I didn't call you. Me: Oh. Took me awhile to re-alize it is not that she has forgotten she called me. She's calling a 25-year-old Dayna who is still on the radio in Houston. I'm the older Dayna that looks like the age she thinks she is now. Again, crazy-ass disease. (Be sure to see the note from Dr. Justiz in the Resources sec-tion of this book.)

Crazy ass it certainly is. Cheers my friend.

Have been though it with my father and wife's grandmother. Pick out the comical moments for later memories and let the crazy ones go.

My grandmother is going through the same thing. One day I am called her sister, the next day she calls me her favorite niece. She knows that I am related to her and that I am her family. She just forgets the particulars.

AUGUST 18, 2014

Someone asked me the other day, "You have such a great attitude about this. Do you ever cry?" In a word, yes. Rivers till it floods. Sometimes it is the smallest thing that sets me off. Walked into Beyond Beaute' Clear

Lake for a massage the other day. Front desk handed me a bag. Inside? Cupcakes made by Kellie Holliday based on the recipe my mom used every year for my birthday cake until last year when she began to forget. Then Suni the Masseuse to the Stars handed me a jar of homemade pickled okra — my mom used to make that every year and I love it. (Fun fact: I was always in trouble for drinking the pickle juice out of the jar before the okra was all gone.) I made it all the way thru the massage and into my car before the floodgates opened. Then I went home and drank the pickle juice.

Dayna, your ability to "cowgirl up" in the face of pain speaks volumes!

Friends who do things like that for others are truly precious gems. I'm sorry you're mom is going through this, and consequently you and your family. Love from friends and family sure help as much as anything can help.

Random acts of kindness are priceless.

August 25, 2014

There are a lot of firsts and lasts with this.
The first time you realize you will never get your special birthday cake from her ever again.
The first time she forgets your name.
The first time she asks how she knows you.
The first time she asks the same question 15 times in less than 15 minutes, "Where is Dack?"
The first time you tell your son to be sure and get a picture because it might be the last. Yeah, that one was hard.

Just answer each and every question with a smile on your face.

61

Oh my, how well I know all of those questions. My dad had it and he did the same thing to my mom, the questions, and the uncertainty of who she was.

My grandmother accused me of stealing from her.

All of those are very difficult and emotionally draining! I so understand ... my mom is at the 6 minute hour ... every 6 minutes we have the same conversation ... heart breaking!

AUGUST 31, 2014

Mom used to spend hours going through her old personal phone books trying to recognize a name. Recently, she's down to one and has thrown the others away. (I retrieved those from the trash so I will have names and numbers at a later date). She rarely looks at the one she saved, she just doesn't know who the names belong to anymore. But ... she knows she had friends and family and a lot of 'em. It is very sad to see the overwhelming number of people who don't bother to keep in touch or reach out in any way. I try to send her a card at least once a week if not more. She loves to get mail and it makes her think people still care.

If you can't get to see someone who is ill or suffering from something like this, at least send a card. Even if they don't remember you! You have no idea what a valuable and meaningful impact a simple card from the grocery store and a stamp will have on someone's well being. Even from a stranger.

Well said and I couldn't agree more. My Mom could hardly speak the last year or so of her life and some people stayed away — just too uncomfortable I guess. Broke my heart for her she loved having visitors right up to her last days.

I lost my Dad to all Heifers last November and my aunt ... his sister in February. It is a hard thing to watch, but know that deep down inside her heart is a place that holds on to all that is precious.

Stupid auto-correct ... LOL ... Alzheimer's

That is the best auto correct ever! We breed and show heifers and I thought my GOD — she lost her Dad to a herd of heifers. That is something you don't hear every day!! LOL

I thought cows killed someone! That is the funniest thing today!!

September 4, 2014

She may be forgetting many things but she remembers Nick and she remembers that for the longest time he only ate peanut butter and jelly sandwiches. Each night, after dinner, Regal Estates Retirement and Assisted Living Community puts out fresh fruit and PBJ sandwiches for the residents in case they get hungry and need a snack. Mom takes all the PBJ sandwiches every night and hoards them for Nick. Thanks to Mom for being such a wonderful grandmother to this day - and - to Regal Estates for looking the other way each evening. Nick makes a big deal out of receiving the large bag of squished sandwiches each time he sees her. Happy 15th birthday to such a fine young man we have raised...

She has always been such a caregiver! One of my favorite childhood memories is leaving your house with my "snack bag" that Aunt Fran packed for the car ride.

When my mother-in-law had Alzheimer's she would tell us to take tampons from the QV club to save money.

63

September 8, 2014

Kristi Hoss Schiller always invites me on the most amazing adventures. I was supposed to be in NYC with her and her organization K9s4Cops.org to ring the opening NASDAQ bell this morning. I cancelled at the last minute because Mom was having a jewelry show at Regal Estates Retirement and Assisted Living Community and I wanted to be there to help. If you have a strand of nice, good pearls from Nazar's in Houston, odds are Mom strung them — she did that for 27 years for them and was sought after for her mastery of pearl stringing. She also had very successful, private jewelry shows all the time. Now, I make the bracelets (poorly) — she thinks she makes them and sells them for bingo money. Yesterday, she was not in the least bit interested or involved. In fact, she really didn't remember that she used to string pearls and she used to tell those stories all the time. Yesterday, there were no stories. Instead, she kept asking when we were going to Dayna's house. I am so glad I stayed home and was able to do this with her. The last jewelry show for Fran's Fine Jewelry was a grand adventure indeed.

> *Wow. The strong emotions I have from reading this can't even begin to compare to the emotions you experience every day. Thank you for sharing this. And yes, I have some Nazar's pearls. I've known him for nearly 30 years. Out of all of the pieces I've collected, I'll be looking at those pearls a lot differently now; I had no idea. Hugs*

> *This brings back many fond memories of Fran's Fine Jewelry shows, which I helped with many times. I think of her every day when I put on my jewelry, most of it I got from Fran! Dayna, you are a wonderful daughter and your mom always said that. This is sad and hard to take and you are doing the best you can. Dack is a good grandson too.*

SEPTEMBER 10, 2014

Mom was great friends' with the late (and missed) Caroline Emel in Quail Valley and thrilled years ago to find out Caroline's son/our friend/former El Lago mayor Brad Emel owned our favorite local diner, the Seabrook Classic Cafe. Over the years, she had delighted in saying hello to Brad and catching up with his family. Over the last year, she has become increasingly obsessed with seeing Brad — or that man at that place — as we have now learned to recently translate. At our most recent lunch, she confided to me, " I think that man is sweet on me." And, she giggled, "I think I'm sweet on him." As we say in Texas, bless your heart Brad for playing along so graciously. You make her day. And, you make her swoon.

What a great guy for going along with it!

How sweet. I remember when we had to gather three neighbors to witness my grandmother signing her will and she flirted outrageously with my neighbor's husband. And when say "flirted," I mean downright bawdy.

Puppy love at its finest!

SEPTEMBER 15, 2014

Thanks to all who dropped by for Mom 's 85th birthday party last week at Regal Estates Retirement and Assisted Living Community. Fran Nicholson was always known for her gift of gab (I come by it honestly). She could talk to anyone about anything at anytime and have a ball doing so. She never met a stranger. Now, she can't remember how to say much and can't comprehend much of what you are saying. She just sort of stares blankly and glances around occasionally. Her conversation is now limited to:

I like you. (She says that to people she recognizes.)

When are you coming to get me? (One of the only things she knows to say to me when she calls.)

I really like this place (when you come to get her and she doesn't want to leave).

Where's that boy? (Dack.)

I have the things for Nick. (Remembers his name and things are PBJ's she takes from the counter each night.)

I have to play bingo. (Get the hell out of my way.)

Oh yeah. (She says that to about everything else.)

Who is this? (How she answers the phone now.)

Out of all the things this disease takes away, not being able to talk to my Mom is the worst. I see her almost every day but I can't share anything with her. The good thing is she still says, "I like you" to me. And I like her, too.

She has a shining spirit!

Dayna, thanks for sharing your memories of your Mom. Mothers are so very special. She is in a very tough stage of life. She is in her own little world and happy in her own way. It is more difficult for you and family because you cannot communicate with her now. But you know what she still has that unconditional love for you. She just can't share it with you at this state she is in. That love never stops that is what makes Mother's so very special. Hang in there you still have her.

September 17, 2014

For a woman who loved to talk, phone calls are now strangely a bad thing. She is having a hard time understanding who is on the phone and what you want. She now often answers the phone with, "Who is this?" If she doesn't recognize your name or voice (which is just about everyone), she says, "I don't want to talk to you" or "I don't know who you are." And hangs up. I have to tell friends and family not to take it personally, just don't call anymore. Personal visits are gold, pure gold. The next best thing is mail. She loves to get mail from anyone. Thanks to everyone who has sent a card, a note small gifts, etc. She carries it all around in her walker and shows the loot to everyone over and over. She just beams.

Mail is very special. A card with lovely flowers can bring a smile for sure.

A loved parent with Alzheimer's is the most difficult thing in the world to go through except for that of a sick child.

I have worked with several Alzheimer's patients as in home care. There are ways to make the best of it. I have found that looking at the past, pictures, cards, etc. can help. If they don't know who they are, you tell them all about them.

SEPTEMBER 21, 2014

There's a story in my first book, "Rock to the Top," about how Mom got her nickname "Flo" — several of her tennis buddies called her that but it wasn't until she got to be close friends with Debbie Beard in Quail Valley that Flo really started to stick. Debbie's husband ZZ Top drummer Frank Beard, took great pleasure in only calling her Flo. Once he started that, it just stuck and everyone did it. Miss Fran became Flo — so she dressed the part for us one Halloween. She was wicked fun!

Kiss my grits!!

Priceless!

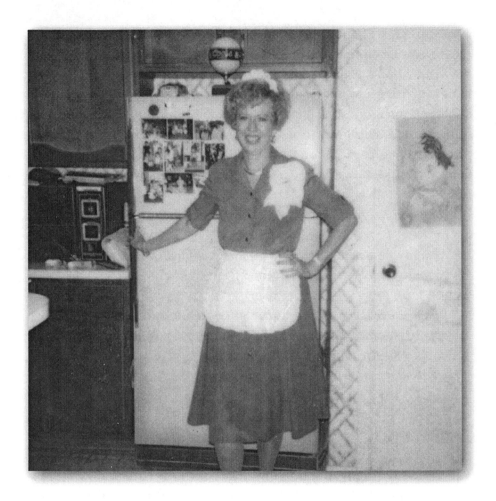

SEPTEMBER 22, 2014

Not many funny stories left but will continue to tell you stories about her wonderful past — and not-so great things you have to do and put up with when a loved one goes through this little adventure. Today it was a call to AT&T Non –Customer- Service. Guess what? When you are incapacitated (Alzheimer's, stroke, coma, paralyzed, dead), your lovely mobile phone contract stays intact or you can cancel and pay a hefty penalty. According to supervisor Camilo this morning, "Can't you just give the phone to someone else in the family?" And let's not forget his, "Well that's too bad but you still have to stay with the contract through April of 2015 or pay a penalty." Oh Camilo, Camilo, Camilo, some really dark humor is bubbling in my brain.

Well, from what I understand, they would disconnect the service and could ruin her credit for 10 years. Would that really be a problem?

What would happen if you didn't pay it? Ruin your mom's credit. It's a service she no longer uses nor can use due to health issues. Stand firm. We can maybe nudge them into changing their "policy."

> Dayna note: It is part of our family share plan. So yes, it would affect my credit.

September 23, 2014

One of the things I love about social media is the past connections you would not have ever found otherwise. Meet Cindi Woods — my best friend from elementary school in Sharpstown, Texas. She moved to Indiana and we lost touch. We picked right up where we left off this weekend when she and her family came to stay with us. It is VERY difficult, but over time I have learned not to say 'Remember' to Mom. She has Alzheimer's! Of course she doesn't remember. When you say the word remember to a memory loss patient, it is very frustrating and maddening for them. Don't do it. I introduced her to Cindi as a longtime friend and showed her the pictures of the shows we used to put on in the backyard. (We charged 25 cents per person.) I was an entrepreneur even then). Mom had a lovely time with Cindi and the Woods' family. She doesn't remember Cindi nor will she remember the visit. Alzheimer's is like having a stranger, a new friend, in the house each visit. Treat them as such and share your life with them. All over again. The third clown is Ellen. We lived on Hendon Lane. Ellen where are you?

Oh I can vouch for the shows. You even charged for a Ritz cracker.

I have often thought of meeting Ms. Fran. I will get there with a friend soon and introduce ourselves. SWEET. New friends.

September 24, 2014

ZZ Top's Dusty Hill fell in the tour bus recently and broke his hip. A nephew due to an undisclosed illness has replaced AC/DC Malcolm Young. Eddie Van Halen has had a hip replacement. So, Mom's new neighbor's name (Jimmy Page) made me laugh yesterday. You're never too old to rock and roll! By the way, when I started doing these, it was just to let friends and family members know what was happening every month. Then you encouraged me to write more, which I appreciate, so I started doing one every other week or so. Then, these posts became cathartic for me. And I increased the frequency to every week. Now, as I see her slipping away so fast, I am posting almost daily. It is as if I can hang on to her just a little bit harder if I just keep writing.

Love your stream of consciousness as you make this painful journey with your Mom. But you got me wrapped around the axle with Dusty's hip fracture and Eddie's replacement. Whiskey Tango Foxtrot ... we ain't old enough yet for that &**$# yet.

Because of you, your Mom is giving each one of us a gift with every post. And it is always a surprise when some tears well up as I smile at the humor you find in all of it. The only thing I recall Voltaire saying, "God is a comedian playing to an audience afraid to laugh." You lead us past that fear and connect in a unique and powerful way.

September 29, 2014

Today's poll! We brought Mom to the house yesterday for dinner as we do every Sunday. She had $36 dollars in her wallet. I give her a couple of dollar bills here and there for bingo but took over all of her finances over a year ago. So, where did it come from? Here are our guesses:
She took it from the church offerings (which by the way I think is an abomination that the church would even take donations from people on a fixed income with memory problems but that's a post for another day).
She is petty criminal, stealing others' purses.
She is turning tricks in her studio apartment.
She (fill in the blank).

She won at bingo?

She's selling your stuff on eBay!

She has a sugar daddy?

October 1, 2014

Me: You are such a great momma
Mom: I'm a momma? (Wide-eyed but smiling.)
Me: Yep. You have a son named Scooter and a daughter, named Dayna.
Mom: Oh yeah, oh yeah. (She repeats that phrase a lot to anything.)
Me: And I AM that daughter Dayna.
Mom: (Whips her head to look at me narrow eyed.) Well then, prove it! (I burst out laughing)
Me: I don't have to, just look at me.
Mom: (With a big smile), You look like me. Oh yeah, oh yeah.
Me: And, I'm the best damn daughter in the whole world.
Mom still smiling: Oh yeah, oh yeah.

71

I want to be named Scooter LOL.

When I tell mine she has 4 kids, she says, Oh Brother. LOL!!

OCTOBER 7, 2014

If you asked me to make a list of the hardest moments through this journey, I never would have thought closing her phone account would be at
the top ...
The phone has become too stressful for her.
When it rings, she says the same thing to all but a hand full of us: Who
is this (no hello)? Why are you calling? I don't want to talk to you. Click.
She just can't understand who it is especially since she doesn't' remem-
ber most people.
She will then proceed to call that person back — 30, 40, 50, even 60
times in a row. Hanging up when she doesn't recognize the voice or
know what to say.
If you include your phone number in a card: She does the same thing.
Or she loses the phone and that becomes a crisis — no matter the hour
of day or night.
She keeps giving away the charging cord because she no longer likes it
and does not want it in her room.
You figure that one out.
So I told her the phone was broken and I needed to have it checked.
That was two weeks ago and she hasn't asked for it back yet. I need to call
AT&T and cancel her account. (I finally found a sympathetic rep). This
is a woman who loved to talk to people. As far back as I can remember
my Mom was on that kitchen phone with the cord stretched across the
room — usually cooking, talking and laughing.
I can't bring myself to make that final call. It seems so, well final.

*Before you turn it off save a recording of her voice mail answer with her
voice ... that is one thing I wish I had done.*

All the "firsts" are so hard. Moving them to a facility, taking the car, dis-connecting the phone, the list goes on ... but she's still here with you. You can see her, make her laugh, hug her, just sit with her and not even talk. I'd give everything to have my mother back for one day. Cherish every second with her. May the stretched cord memories live on!

October 8, 2014

Mom has started throwing away her socks and underwear. She no longer likes them. I can't say I blame her.

Commando baby! TMI?

Get that feisty woman some Hanky Panky Thongs.

I put in my medical directive/will that as long as I was enjoying myself, whether or not I had dementia, that I did not want care withheld. Who knows what happens in the unconscious. Maybe we have many persons in there. Your Mom seems joyful despite her illness and confusion. That should be a blessing to you. Follow HER joy!!!

Wheeeee!

October 12, 2014

Miss Fran, smile!
No, it will make my hair gray.
Mom was always so proud, even bragging about the fact she did not have gray hair.
Her hair stayed brown (with 'natural' blonde highlights) until almost a year ago.
The more the gray started to appear the more she avoided mirrors.

It's interesting the mirror in the bathroom does not bother her — because that is where we all look our worst early in the morning after rising. So, she'll look then with no problem but avoids them the rest of the day, even becoming visibly upset sometimes when she walks past a mirror. It took a while to figure out what it was, but it is the gray hair bothering her.

As the disease progresses, many patients have crazy perceptions of things, many become paranoid — such as the people in the TV are coming to get me, etc. Mom's problem is she doesn't like or recognize the old woman in the mirror. And brown highlights are out of the question — she can't sit still that long and would probably be too drastic of a change at this point. So I need to start telling her things like:

I love your hair color.

It's not gray. It's beautiful silver.

You look like a Queen with that beautiful hair.

We are going to call you Queen Mimi.

Your ideas?

My mother doesn't recognize herself in the mirror, and thinks she is looking at her mother. I think what you're doing by telling her positive things about her hair color are perfect.

I think distraction is the key, for the time being. My Mom was obsessed with money, particularly coins. Until she started to eat them!

Brings back so many very emotional memories, just being there is so important for her and even more for you. As I read these posts I remember like it was yesterday with my mom's final months, when I would leave and wonder why — and if she really knew who I was. But I would do it again over many times without hesitation. All of these things you share about, wow, I wish there was social media back then. I never liked the answers doctors gave and I learned more from the few with similar issues, the emotion running down my cheeks now are for the wonderful person you are and the incredible strength you show daily helping your mom and all you do.

October 14, 2014

It dawned on me recently that Mom has forgotten how to hug. She was a great hugger. Now, she just sort of puts one arm around you and kind of pats. So the last few visits, we have had hugging lessons. I laugh and tell her 'that was a lousy hug — try again.' We practice 'til she puts both arms around me and holds me tight. Here she is teaching the lesson to her dog Sandy. Next lesson will be to hold that pose for 10 seconds. Then we will work on more. I don't want her to ever let go ...

> *Your journey with her, albeit heartbreaking at times, is an amazing one and a true testament of the love between a mother and her child.*
>
> *Your journey opened my heart to feelings I need to address.*
>
> *The last line got me. Treasure each day and hug!*
>
> *Reading this made me cry. When I saw her hugging her dog, I smiled.*
>
> *I am so grateful for these posts, and I am reading the 36 Hour Day on your advice. Your "ministry" brings much strength and comfort to many, and I hope to you as well.*
>
> **See the image on the next page.*

Dayna note: Just for the record, this is the first one I've written where I actually cried as I wrote it.

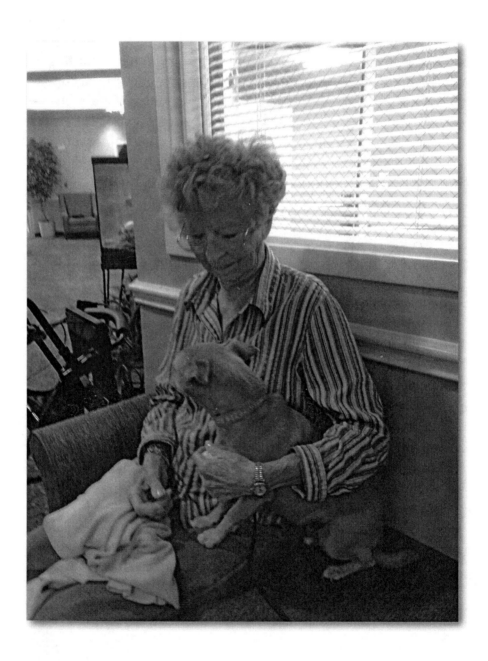

OCTOBER 19, 2014

I bought this pillow years ago at Paula Fridkin's shop in the River Oaks Shopping Center. My mother has never liked it. The other day she started giggling. I asked her what was so funny? She pointed at the pillow and said " Now that's funny." Oh yeah, Mom, Oh yeah.

I've been quoting that pillow for years

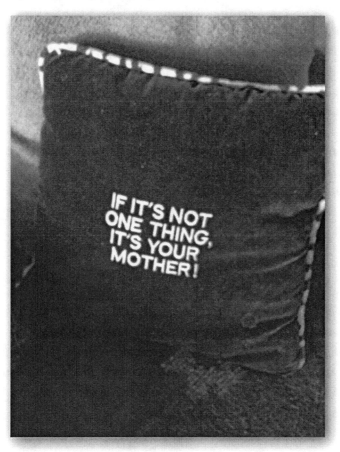

OCTOBER 21, 2014

Want to get mad about a disease that is spreading like wildfire across the country and killing many?

A HazMat suit won't help you on this one.

No blood transfusion will cure you.

There is no cure available. Yet.

It is inevitable your life will be touched by it.

One in six people will be diagnosed with Alzheimer's.

50 percent of people 85 or older will be diagnosed with Alzheimer's.

Alzheimer's is 100 percent fatal.

Elder long-term care will bankrupt most families.

500,000 people die a year of Alzheimer's.

If I can scare just one of you into investing in Long Term Care Insurance, I will have done my job. Do it now, I don't care what your age is.

Your phone and cable cost more. Get your priorities straight right now.

Before it is too late.

Get scared and get mad about Alzheimer's.

(See the Long-term Care Insurance section in the Resources section of this book.)

Thank you, good info to know. I have to take action!

I love my stepfather like he is a biological dad. I can't get over him cancel-ing the long-term care insurance when he knew mother was sick. I have to swallow my rage every day when he bitches about all of the work he has to do to take care of Mom. It's a really screwed situation, and he single handedly made a detrimental choice that has made a catastrophic event much worse. My Mother deserves better.

Absolute best time to buy long- term care insurance is in your 30's. The earlier you do it,
the cheaper it is!

OCTOBER 22, 2014

Dirty little family secret. Mom hates old people. Always has. Just never had patience for walkers, wheelchairs, etc. As the disease started to take hold, her filters have slowly but surely gone. First she would mumble under her breath. Then, after she moved to Assisted Living, she started saying out loud, "Look at all these old people. They should just get out of that wheelchair and walk." In the last year, Mom's brown hair turned silver (not bad for 85) and she started using a walker. We aren't that far off from a wheelchair. Yet, she still complains about the old people she is surrounded by. And, now we have a new trick. If someone in a wheelchair isn't moving fast enough in front of her, she rams it continuously with her walker, smiling sweetly all the while, not having a clue this is wrong. And let someone try to pass beside her on their walker, Mom turns into Jeff Gordon, ramming wheels and making the pass. I know it's wrong. But it's funny. You just have to be there. BTW, there is a woman she exchanges verbal smack downs with all day. Made them sit on either side of me and smile. All the while, both are saying nasty remarks about each other. I can't wait until what is left of my filter is gone.

Go Flo Go.

I think those kinds of rivalries and feuds are fairly common in nursing/ rehab/seniors centers. A friend of ours had to bring his dad home for home care, because, he got kicked out of a center for picking fights and being aggressive. They look like they are in good shape; I just don't want to see them wrestle.

OMG: I remember when my Mom's filter started going. I took her to lunch at a little strip-center cafe and a full-figured gal walked in. My mother said, "Well, it doesn't look like she needs ANY lunch!" After making sure the woman hadn't heard her (she was close enough that she could have), I just cracked up.

I remember this well! My mom learned a bunch of curse words that she had never, ever used before and didn't see a problem with it!

When Mother was in the nursing home a sweet looking little old lady passed by her and as she passed she said Bitch. I nearly died. I was afraid to leave her there.

Did you ever have a filter to start?

Dayna note: I was waiting for that comment from someone.

OCTOBER 28, 2014

I have talked to my mom almost every morning since the day I left for college. It was just our thing. I had to take her phone away a few weeks ago — I posted about that. This morning I was on my way to a meeting downtown when I realized how much I missed that daily morning conversation. I called Regal Estates to ask if they would have her call me.

And I fell completely apart on the phone with the receptionist (so sorry Lauren). They did have Mom call me a few minutes later and I was grateful to hear her voice. A few hours later I got an email from Marie in the front office making sure I was okay. That started it all over again. (It's okay Marie.)

Having you follow along on this journey gives me so much strength and I thought hard about you as I tried to stop crying. I have found lots of humor and will continue to find more. But today I found a deep well of tears I had no idea was getting ready to overflow. And, here comes the waterworks again … thanks for being here with me.

It is my pleasure to take this journey with you. No apologies necessary. The emotions were to take control at some point in time. You have the largest support group I know!

Thank you for letting us follow this journey with you. You are expressing the words and emotions of many and it is a comfort to others to know they are not alone.

Thank you for sharing this journey with us, and making it okay, (or at least not so incredibly terrifying). You are modeling how to continue the relationship with one you love so dearly. You are giving back as much support as you are getting (((((Hugs)))))

OCTOBER 30, 2014

Need to find someone? Meeting with someone new? A world and wealth of information is at your fingertips with a little amateur sleuthing on your part. Each morning I write a success tip. Every afternoon or so, it gets personal and I write an update about my journey with Mom and Alzheimer's. Today the two are combined. Going through her old photo albums, I found my long lost 'sister' Amor. Amor was a young nursing student from the Philippines that our family hosted in the 60's. I found a picture yesterday of Mom visiting Amor and her family in the 80's in Montreal. It took me about 30 minutes but with Google, a location and the names of her husband and kids, I was able to find one of her sons on Facebook and find an email address for him through one of the websites. I reached out with the pictures and he replied back, copying mom — Amor. She and I had a lovely, teary conversation last night. I think I feel a trip to Montreal coming on — anyone need a speaker in Quebec.

I love modern technology. But I love these updates even more!!! Stay strong!

NOVEMBER 9, 2014

As people learn of Mom's diagnosis, these words come up again and again. She was always so: thoughtful, fun-loving, kind, friendly, sweet. Well, a mean streak is starting to emerge. What started as somewhat humorous is now becoming a problem, a danger to others. For example: she is mad at the man across the hall because he won't close his door, drives her crazy. So, she hit him in the leg with her walker the other day. Granted he shook his finger at her, and said, "Stop yelling at me." So she rammed his leg. Sigh. We had this talk yesterday:

Me: Mom, you must stop hitting people with your walker.

Mom: I didn't hit anyone.

Me: Mom, you did.

Mom: What are you talking about? I don't hit people with my walker.

Me: Mom, they say you did.

Mom: God Damn It! I didn't hit anyone.

Me: Mom they said they saw you do it.

Mom: They are lying.

Me: Mom, you can't do this.

Mom: I do NOT hit people with my walker.

Me: Mom, I've seen you do it to a few other people.

Mom: (pauses, contemplates) You have?

Me: Yes, Mom. I saw you ram that woman's wheelchair because she wasn't moving fast enough for you.

Mom: Ok, well maybe there have been a few ...

Had to bite the inside of my cheek to keep from laughing out loud.

> *Alzheimer's is such an insidious disease, robbing a person of their mental faculties and understanding of their surroundings and interactions with it. This incident is quite typical. Even the gentlest and kindest Alzheimer's patient can lash out at those around them in frustration, then completely forget what they have done a moment later. At least your mom has good care. All you can do is show them that you care, over and over again.*

My dad took a guy's painting out of his room. I will never forget what he told me when I walked in to visit him and he was standing there holding it. He said that he got it from a garage sale. His exact words were, I kid you not, were, "I got this off this old guy." I was just dying inside with laughter.

My Mama suddenly hurled F Bombs at everyone. She would flip off the grandkids. It's been 4 years since she left but at the time it was shocking. You are not alone. I pray for you all D.

I just can't click LIKE to posts like this ...

Dayna note: This is serious now that she has started to put others in danger. We will have to move her to a memory care unit in the next couple of weeks. I am touring several over the next few days. I was hoping we had a few more months with the wonderful people at Regal Estates Retirement and Assisted Living Community. Thanks to Bonnie Pate Schoellkopf and the entire staff for all they do.

NOVEMBER 11, 2014

Mom no longer looks at photo albums. It upsets her because she doesn't recognize anyone, even her younger self. And, she thinks all the pictures of me are of her. Which is understandable. There are many where we could be twins. I am digitizing all her old pictures so I will always have them. Came across this one. Growing up, Mom adopted every living creature — from stray animals and ducks in the lake to teenagers who had runaway to visiting Wimbledon champion tennis players. She would invite anyone and everyone for dinner or to stay for a night or more. Oh yeah, I come by it honestly.

Maybe you can show pictures to her and just talk about how wonderful that person is for caring. If she asks, say it is her. And say the photo was taken when she was young so it is understandable she didn't recognize it. Then talk about what you remember all the wonderful things she did for all even if she doesn't.

It is good to know she lived life to the fullest.

She had a rich and full life. Nothing can take that away from her.

What a beautiful picture.

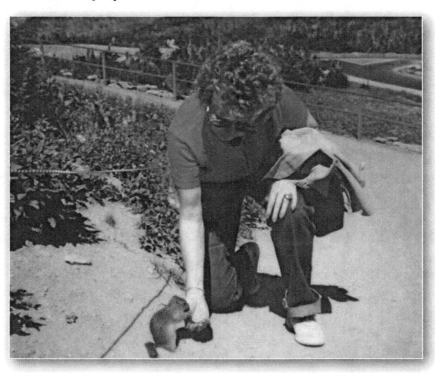

NOVEMBER 13, 2014

This is the update ...

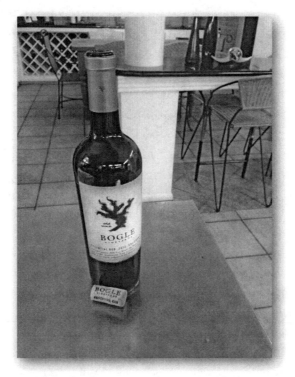

Everything is a little better with wine. Just saying ...

Nuff said. A little caregiver burnout, eh?

The only thing missing is the straw.

NOVEMBER 17, 2014

Yes, I hit a caregiver wall late last week. Yep, full speed and no brakes into that wall. Thanks to all who saw the bottle of wine pic and figured that out. Your support, calls, emails, comments, and general comforting were — well — comforting. I took a break the rest of the weekend. I just had to. That's one of the hardest things to do — to back away and take some time to take care of yourself. We are fortunate that we can afford to have mom in a place where she is well taken care of when I need a few mental health days. MOST are not so fortunate and I have no idea how they do it. Are you a family member or good friend, maybe the sibling who never visits or just visits occasionally for a few minutes? Offer to take a week and do all the visiting, shopping, doctor's visits, everything that has to be done in a situation like this. And offer to do it every six weeks or so. Give the caregiver a break. Thanks to my wonderful children and bonus daughter who spent some time with mom over the weekend. She was so happy. And, I got a chance to breathe. (And to my wonderful Aunt Mary and Uncle Jim who see her every Sunday without fail.)

Being a caretaker is a rewarding experience but is so hard at times. You are glad you can do it, but at the same time you get both physically and emotionally tired. And it is often a private battle that no one who hasn't done it can truly understand. Here is to all of those who have been down this road. We need to lean on those like us for sanity's sake and Dayna's daily posts have offered a forum. Keep up the good work Dayna. I know you are tired but your mom appreciates it and that is priceless, even though she e can't show it at this time.

Hugs! Put your own oxygen mask on first. Hard to do but necessary!

I'm glad I read this twice. The first time, I read that you hit a caregiver!

November 23, 2014

I am a firm believer in speaking up and asking for what you need or want. For some reason, I have found that hard when it comes to Mom.

I feel guilty asking others to participate and help, visit, etc. But I have learned you have to get over that and just ask. If people can help, they will. If they can't, they let me know and hopefully don't feel guilty. I hope those that I ask know it is because of my love for them and our much-appreciated friendship that I can even begin to ask — no matter the answer. Then there is Cheryl Evans who has made visiting a part of her routine whether I ask or not. That is a true friend — she and Mija who endures many wardrobe changes for the cause ...

I didn't know Fran had Alzheimer's. I'm glad a mutual friend shared this on my wall. I used to work for her in high school stringing beads! I'm so sorry to hear that she is going through this struggle. Thankfully she has a supportive family and she looks absolutely lovely.

November 26, 2014

We are in Miami for Thanksgiving. A hard decision to make, but I need to take care of all family members, not just Mom. She is in a fabulous place, Regal Estates in League City. We are moving Mom soon because the disease is progressing past what the incredible caregivers at Regal Estates can do for her and us. She will move to equally great caregivers at Brookdale Ellington. We visit, family and friends visit, even complete strangers visit Mom. There are however residents in both facilities who rarely have visitors, no one ever comes by. This week and every week, be thankful for your elderly family and friends — and let them know you care.

When my dad was in the hospice there was a sad old lady there that I would talk to when I came to visit. She passed the same weekend as my dad. Her two daughters came to collect her things — no one knew who they were, they had never come to see her. Another lady had a lot of family visit and was always happy. I'd sit with her for a while when I came and every visit ended with us getting engaged to be married. Her name was Mildred.

My Mom was in a facility when I could no longer care for her. There were so many that had loving families around ... and so many that were just dumped there. It is so damn sad to see.

This I will tell you, my wife's dad we went and saw every week, my mom we go and see twice a week, the more involved you are in any facility the better care they get.

If YOU want to be taken care of when you are old, then take care of your parents when they are old. Your kids are going to learn from your example.

NOVEMBER 29, 2014

This is what helps when you come home from a long trip, you're facing changes with mom, and you know the next couple of weeks are going to be rough. Then you find cards in your mailbox from friends. Know a caregiver? Send them a smile and a hug anyway you can.

On our third round through this forest! Different each time, take care of yourself that's life.

I just went through some changes with mine too. Luckily the staff wears the same gear as the hospitals so she keeps the idea she has to do what they want. What drives me nuts is she asks to see my brothers, I get them there ... and she tells them to leave her room. Lol. And now, her room-mate with the same first name says the same thing. GET OUT NOW! It's hilarious when they do it unison! Lol

December 1, 2014

Got Mom all packed up and ready for her move to a new place with more assistance and eventually memory care and hospice. She was over for a few hours late yesterday. As we were packing her up to go off with my aunt and uncle, I said to Charlie, " I'm so tired of her." I could not believe the words came out of my mouth but they did. I think most caregivers want to say something like that occasionally but are in fear of what others will think. Having lost my filter years ago (thanks KLOL), I will tell you I said it. I'm not proud of it but it is the truth. Sometimes I hate this person who has taken over my time, my energy, my Mom. Thank you to Trace Manchaca for the angel you sent her. I have tied it to Mom's walker as a reminder that she is my angel and I am doing the best I can …

For those of us who have been caregivers, we understand. Reading your posts, through tears, anger, and laughter… we applaud you for being so honest and devoted. Perfect is asking too much, you are true and human. Hang in there!

It is mentally and emotionally exhausting to be a caregiver on a daily basis. And sometimes frustrating when the person you love has changed from independent to dependent. Remember to take some time for YOU and lean on your support system.

It's like being on the frontlines of a long battle.

But soldiers survive, so can we.

As I was sitting at the nursing home yesterday for my daily visit with my mother-in-law, I was thankful I had not visible "thought bubbles" over my head like in a cartoon. This disease is the "long goodbye" and some days are just a bitch! Thank you for your honesty. It feels strange to hold the tensions of "I love this person but I am so sick of doing this."

December 5, 2014

Mom worked with the top jewelers in Houston, specifically stringing high-end pearls for Nazar's. She loved her work (she was one of the best in the country) and loved her jewelry. Now she only remembers each day to put on the bracelets I made her. She goes nowhere without those which is very sweet. Moving her the other day, I found one earring on the floor, not sure what she did with the other one. Just one sad little earring, from a woman who always had on her jewelry!

My sister said mom left a note behind with her symptoms. Breaks my heart each time I think of it.

Your mom took her bracelets off and handed them to me, and I said, "are these for me?" she said "no, those are Dayna's, give them back!" LOL!

December 7, 2014

One of the hardest things to do when you lose someone is finally make that decision to go through their things, saving a few and getting rid of the rest. Here is something you don't read about or hear about — at least I haven't. I moved Mom three times so far. And will do it one more time in the next few months to the Memory care side of Brookdale. Each time, I have to relive all the memories and then get rid of a few more pieces of her life — pictures, clothes, collectibles, and keepsakes. She doesn't know what it is, doesn't want it, and I hate stuff. This to me, is so far one of the worst things about this long goodbye. Each time I move her, pieces of her life are whittled down to even less.

*Anyone want to buy a Lalique glass bowl?

This is truly one of the hardest jobs you will go through ... all the memories, and treasures will bring smiles, laughter and tears! It will change the way you look at possessions. My thoughts and prayers are being sent your way.

I would like the bowl.

I never know what to say and clicking the Like button doesn't seem right. I wish there was an I'm-thinking-of-you-as-you-go-through-this-pain button.

Put the nice pieces up on eBay and donate the proceeds to Alzheimer's research (or to her nursing home if it's a nonprofit).

DECEMBER 16, 2014

People often ask me if Mom recognizes/knows me. Yes and no. It's really not that black and white with this crazy disease. She recognizes me and is very happy to see me. She tells everyone I am her daughter. She tells me I am a good daughter to her. Then she'll turn right around and ask Charlie if her daughter Dayna knows where her new apartment is. Or, I'll call her and ask what she is doing. She'll tell me her daughter Dayna is coming to visit even though I have just said "Hi Mom, It's Dayna." Again, it is not black and white but the best way I can describe it is there are two of me — the one she sees all the time and the one most vivid in her memory — that one is about 30 and is still on the radio. That's when you learn not to argue and just say yes. And, if you are just a touch wicked, you say, "Isn't Dayna the best?".

It's amazing that you are sharing the experience with us. It's a fascinating insight into a horrible illness.

You do have a great sense of humor! Oddly enough, a friend of mine from ATL told me she met you in NYC at a bar!!

DECEMBER 26, 2014

Mom: Who is that man?
Me: That's Cris, my stepson.
Mom: Is he in the family?
Me: Yes
Mom: I like him.
Me: Me too

At least she likes him!

Thanks for sharing. A lighter moment! Happy New Year!

DECEMBER 29, 2014

There may be a flurry of these updates coming. Mom is changing so fast. I constantly question if I am doing the right thing for her — in so many ways. For example, yesterday I grappled with should I keep bringing her to my house or not? Then, I caught her head just before it hit the tile last night. I glanced up while cooking and saw her teetering on the steps to the kitchen, I flew like superwoman across the kitchen and fell with her, cradling her in my arms with my hand behind her head. Like I've done with my kids when they were little. Then there is the anger. Lots of anger — from her and from other residents. Even with the most advanced Alzheimer's or dementia, I think somewhere in that brain you know you are in a situation you never imagined. Dad was mad with dementia. Mom is mad with her journey. Other residents are angry as well all the time; one even lashed out at Mom today and slapped her. I can't get mad at the facility, it just happens. Last night I was helping Mom in the bathroom (a story for another night). As we washed her hands, I said, "Look at those two lovely ladies in the mirror." She got mad, really mad and pointed at herself, sternly saying, "Tell her to leave. I don't like her. Leave, leave!" She was mad, really mad. I was sad, so sad.

There is nothing more frustrating than trying to help someone who doesn't understand you are trying to help. Especially someone you love so very, very much.

When she lost her speech skills she was so angry and we would all tell her we still loved her as often as we could. Eventually I think, or believe, she came to accept this as normal. She learned to communicate through headshakes and facial expressions.

This story breaks my heart. I will be calling my own mother now. It scares me because I see in her some of the things you are experiencing. I hope you know how many people your journey has touched.

My grandfather had Alzheimer's. One time when I visited him, he punched me in the chest. The punch didn't hurt, but emotionally it hurt like hell.

December 30, 2014

I gave her a photo book and a large stack of photos to choose from. This is her favorite. She shows it to everyone and says, "That's my Dayna." Then she adds, "She never comes to visit."

My sister and I get that all the time now even though we each visit her regularly. It's just part of this crappy disease.

Girlfriend, we are in the same boat. My mom does this also. Thanks for posting. It makes me laugh out loud for real.

ALL Moms say that!

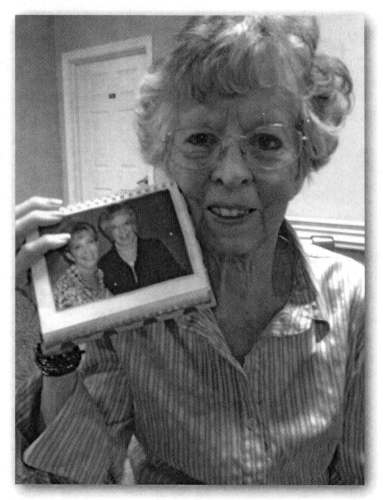

The more it hurts, the more you need to use it in a book.
- Brad Meltzer, best-selling author

2015:

THE LONG GOODBYE

JANUARY 1, 2015

Have done so many of these now; I don't remember if I ever shared this with you. Mom has always hated this pillow, mildly chuckling while seething inside for years. She spent all this past Christmas Day, picking it up and laughing at it.

You could sell those pillows!

Laughter is good.

> Dayna note: I had shared this earlier. See the picture of the pillow on the update for October 19, 2014.

JANUARY 4, 2015

When Mom needs something or is bothered by something, she writes a note. We are note takers and list makers –— I come by this honestly as well. Except now, she writes it over and over. I find dozens of notes around her room on whatever subject she is fixated on — it could be that she needs toothpaste or a meal she wants or any number of things. If I had not seen her do this with me in a mirror last week, I would have thought there was another resident (or staff member) coming into her room and bothering her. I found 12 of these notes the other day. She wants this lady to leave her alone, to get out of her room and stop staring at her. It is her own reflection she is seeing in the mirror. We have told her to do what she can to tolerate this woman. She is actually very nice and just wants to be friends …

I haven't had anyone go through this, but I've become more knowledgeable on the subject thanks to you.

Hang a family picture of her playing tennis over it.

I wonder if you could convince her to smile at "that lady" and see if "that lady" smiling back might suggest that she is kind …

I just hate that she doesn't like the "Lady in the Mirror." I liked the idea of telling her to smile and that maybe when the lady smiles back she will like her then.

January 5, 2015

The Woman in the Mirror Part Two — Took Mom dinner and her dog last night — Charlie, the boys and me. We had a lovely visit. And a long talk about this woman who won't leave (her image in the mirror). We all talked about how nice the woman is and that she just wants to be friends. Mom is very concerned she isn't paying rentJ). Told her I would cover that. Then she added, "She's much older than me."

Start leaving an envelope that says rent payment. Maybe if she thinks the lady should stay if she pays. Just a thought.

Dayna, my former mother-in-law died of Alzheimer's. I remember hearing about the "Mirror" and the fear that can be involved. She went through many of these stages and her daughters should follow your documentation of your mother's disease.

Go Miss Fran! Make that lady pay! Hugs to you. XO

My father told me today that man is crowding his space and putting words in his brain.

My Dad got mad at me for moving the walls.

Dayna note: I said to Wonder Husband last night: This is probably something that should make me sad, but it doesn't. I am absolutely fascinated with this development.

JANUARY 6, 2015

Even crazy women need their nails done. I should know …

I hope the woman in the mirror is not wearing the same color.

My Mom totally loved getting her nails done. She couldn't remember much, but she COULD tell that it was time for a manicure!

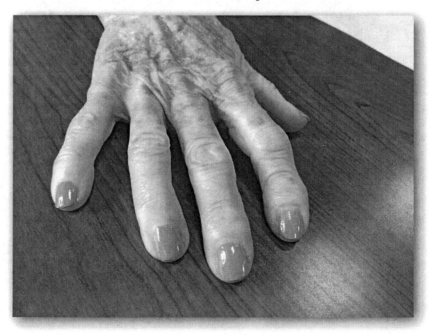

JANUARY 8, 2015

I have tried to get Mom to cut her hair and quit poofing it for 30 years. She finally let them do her hair this week. And she has forgotten that she wears glasses (even though she didn't need them after cataract surgery, they were clear glass). I love the new look, she looks cute and perky and feisty! That said, it took me awhile to figure out why I was a little off last night, a little sad. Then it hit me — she doesn't look like my Mom anymore.

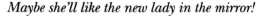

Looks like mom, the one with spunk, the brave adventurous mom. The one you've modeled yourself after.

Maybe she'll like the new lady in the mirror!

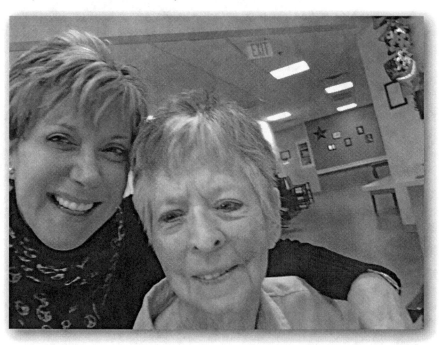

JANUARY 10, 2015

I've told my kids when I turn 75 I want a carton of Marlboro Reds for my birthday. And then I want everyone to back off and let me smoke again. I figure if you get to that point, what the hell! Mom? Never Smoked. Drank only occasionally. But that woman loves to gamble. Used to be trips to Louisiana to play the slots. Then it was Texas Lottery cards. Now, it's Bingo. Not sure she has a clue, but she's happy. However, her only problem with it is the stakes are too low.

> *I really enjoy getting to know your Mom through your updates. She is my kind of woman.*
> *My friends' father has Alzheimer's. He was never a drinker. Not even close! He asked his wife today if he was a wine-o!*
>
> *I remember her showing me how to play slots. We walked in, she gave me my lesson, first pull — she won $300, she was done for the day!*

JANUARY 12, 2015

I check the notes in her room every visit. They are usually things she needs or actions like to get rid of the woman in the mirror. These took my breath away this week. I even considered hiding them not only from you but from Wonder Husband, sons, and brother as well, like I could pretend I didn't find them. Intellectually I know they are about the daughter that comes to visit. Not me — they are about the 35 year old Dayna in the pictures, the Dayna she thinks she is talking to on the phone. The notes did however devastate me emotionally. There is no longer any way to teach her that I AM Dayna. All I can do is cry real hard for a few minutes, drink a glass of wine and be the best Dayna I can for her, whoever that is ...

Another day, another challenge. Chin up! Pop a cork. Move on ...

It's frustrating for a reader to look at someone else's story when the really difficult parts are left out. This is one of those parts ... so, so awful, yet so important to be able to share.

It's eerie. I went through something like this with my Dad on Christmas. Your mind tells you that it's not really your parent but the illness ravaging their very existence. But, it still shakes your heart to the core when you hear the actual hateful words. Through the pain, I send you my love and prayers.

Nothing is more devastating then not being recognized or remembered. Mom often believes she works for the lady that owns this house ... who works her to death and never pays her. She tells me I remind her of her daughter Lisa and asks me all the time if I am "that lady." I am the lady who owns the house. I am her daughter. Her Lisa. It's so sad and does hurt! Just know you are not alone!

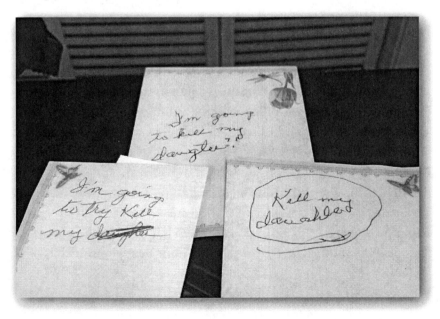

January 16, 2015

Here is what we did to get rid of that pesky "woman in the mirror" — yes the one who wasn't paying rent. Seems to have done the trick — also got rid of all other mirrors in the room. New problem? She's beating on the glass on pictures in the hallways because now she sees her reflection in those. Stay tuned …

A very creative way of problem solving!

I think I'll do this at my house. I'm not so thrilled with the woman in my mirror either!

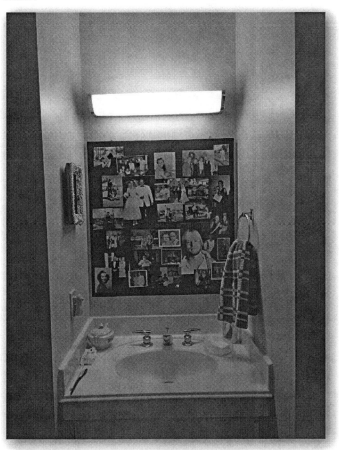

January 18, 2015

The little things that make Mom happy now:
Her dog Sandy.
A ride in the car.
Gumbo from the Seabrook Classic Cafe.
Hiding other residents' walkers in her room.
This shouldn't crack me up but it does. She's like an elderly car thief …

Laugh when you can. It doesn't get any better.

Good for her. Spunk keeps her going.

We have to laugh, so we don't cry. So I did it — out loud.

My mother had a roommate that kept stealing the teeth of everyone. If you had them in the cleaner, she'd come find them and go hide them in various places in other rooms. You never knew where you were going to find false teeth. In pockets of clothes in closets, in eyeglass holders, sometimes she'd put them under pillows. It was a hilarious circus for a while. LOL!

January 24, 2015

Guilt: noun: a bad feeling caused by knowing or thinking that you have done something bad or wrong.
It doesn't matter if you visit every day or once a month. It is all the same to someone in memory care. So, I have to remind myself that I have her in a place that is taking care of her and that is what I am paying for -— peace of mind. I don't have to be there every day. I can't be there every day. I have a husband, sons, friends, and a career not to mention me. All of these people and things need to be taken care of on a regular basis.

106

So, I visit once during the week for lunch if I am not traveling. And, I come on Saturday mornings with her dog Sandy. This morning I also brought a stuffed Sandy doppelganger. She seemed pleased. Sandy? Not so much.

Guilt: noun: a bad feeling caused by not being there every day for someone who was there for me every day.

Guilt should not displace the moment that you share when you visit. You're there other times in mind and spirit. It was the same with my mother. It's sometimes a balancing act. Love conquers all.

If she was "of sound mind" she might make you feel guilty about being there 'only' once/twice a week. But I'm guessing not. She would say, go live your life. Keep your career. Spend time with your lovely husband and children. Don't give up everything for her. I bet that's what she would say and be happy for you.

Besides, you cannot have mother guilt — you aren't Jewish;)

January 29, 2015

A beautiful day for a walk with a dog ... problem with the selfie is the same problem with the mirror. When we take the picture, she is mad "that woman who doesn't pay rent" is in the picture with her dog and her daughter. The picture I show her afterwards is perfectly okay. That's why I can't get her to smile in a selfie. That, or she thinks they are as ridiculous as many of us do but won't say.

Mom is very skeptical of the selfie.

Oh my mother-in-law called tonight to see how "her husband"(my husband) was doing. You are doing good, my friend. Drink wine ... lots of wine!!

107

That woman may not be paying rent, but she's lovely. I love her steely gaze in this one.

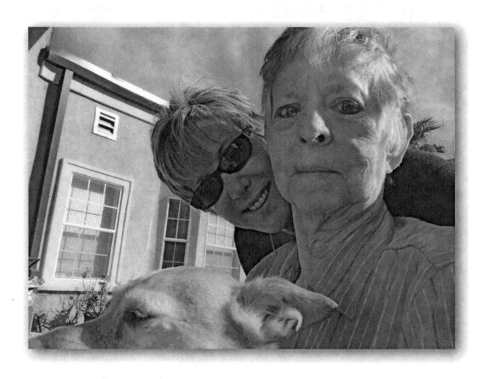

FEBRUARY 4, 2015

At Houston Methodist St. Johns. What dog? I would never sneak a dog into a hospital.

Why it's a therapy dog! Yes it is!!!

A hip flask would have been easier.

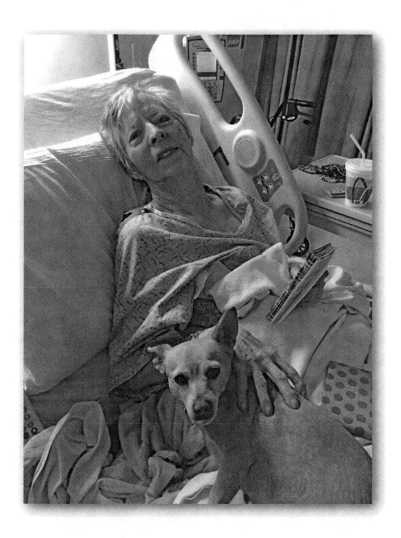

February 4, 2015 (part 2)

Mom had a good night last night. Slept thru the night. Cheryl Evans and her trusty sidekick Mija will be visiting this morning. Family members are dropping by to help throughout the day — much needed so I can take care of the future. There will be discussions with paid caregivers today about the fact she was severely dehydrated and had probably been suffering with the UTI for sometime — something trained caregivers should have easily smelled.

Your Mom's caregiver's should have caught the dehydration, I would think. Maybe your Mom likes Popsicles or other slushy fruit drinks. It may allow her to intake more liquids, as water is so dull. Maybe some color or flavoring could be added to water. Decaf iced tea. Also fruit smoothies.

Also, a note many older folks lose their sense of smell and taste so then nothing is really palatable.

As a nurse I may not have been perfect but I was always certainly well informed and up to date with the specialty area I was working in. I would most certainly be having a discussion with her caregivers, plus I would want information on their qualifications and training in the care of patients with Alzheimer's disease. Sadly as with many things in life the true facts are not always presented. Thinking of both of you.

> Dayna note: If someone in your family or circle of friends is the principle caregiver for someone with Alzheimer's or dementia (or anything like that), OFFER TO HELP AND DO IT. It makes all the difference in the world being able to get things done or rest while someone else takes over the duties for a bit.

FEBRUARY 5, 2015

We had a good day. She's walking and eating well. She had a few visitors (dogs). She told me last night she was going to die soon. I asked her if she was scared and she said, "a little." We talked about all the family she might see. Then I asked her, "Will it be tonight?" "No." "Okay, well then,

I'm going home and will see you tomorrow." "Ok." And there she was waiting for me this morning.

It's definitely okay to think that way. My dad was very sick for 15 years before he died. It's okay to not want to see them suffer anymore.

It's the longest goodbye, isn't it?

You made me feel better. When my husband was dying I just wanted it over and then when he was gone I felt such guilt for thinking that. We never want them gone but sometimes it looks easier for everyone especially the one we are losing. Thank you for sharing.

FEBRUARY 8, 2015

Mom is back in her memory care unit, this time with drugs to keep her calm as needed. Hard to do that for someone who has never been sick before all this and never took so much as an aspirin. Yesterday afternoon she looked at me and asked, "When is Dayna coming?" I said, "I'm Dayna." That causes much confusion. I need to learn to say, "Dayna loves you so much." As she loses more memory, she throws away things in her room she doesn't recognize. (We both hate clutter). One thing she hasn't thrown away is a huge stack of press clippings of mine from high school 'till about a year ago. She sits and goes through those and shows them off to anyone who will look. It used to embarrass me so much when she would ask anyone, anywhere, "Do you know Dayna Steele? Well, this is her." Now, I see what joy it brought her. I've decided she is the Ultimate SteeleWorker.

Your Mom is still there. The wiring just misfires. You indeed are important to her. In the end, that is all that matters.

The Original Steele Worker ...

FEBRUARY 15, 2015

Dropped by with her Valentine present — first time she wasn't all that interested in me. Took her a while to warm up to showing me any attention. Of course, when I got there, she had a lovely red walker for Valentine's Day and I had to pry it from her hands and give it back to the woman it belonged to ... Before I left, I gave her the card and a new red Valentine bracelet. She smiled and said, " You're a good friend." Ok. I'll take that.

I went to see Mother one day and she had on someone else's glasses and we had to look around to find hers on someone else. It never ends ... LOL

Be sure they are keeping her hydrated. Only a little dehydration can have dramatic effects.

We become our parents' best friends as we (become) the ones who tend to their needs no matter the circumstance.

FEBRUARY 22, 2015

Spent the weekend going through mom's recent medical paperwork and another stack of different things I've taken from her apartment. She's throwing away things she doesn't recognize so I've tried to save most of it in case there is anything important or a keepsake. All of her phone books — and there are six — look like this. As she started to forget people, she would cross out their names. Then, as the disease progressed, she started to scratch out the names even harder, followed by tearing out entire pages when she no longer recognized anyone on the page and through the entire page away. I'm going through and trying to keep a record of names of people I know and phone numbers. When the time comes ...

I would have never known to expect it unless someone (you) brought it into my frame of reference.

I'll never forget going through my mother's drawers for her final move. She had hidden Kleenex in the toes of her pantyhose ... hundreds of little bits, visible evidence of her paranoia as she struggled to gain control. She probably threw away her valuables as she retained the Kleenex. So very sad.

This disease is so unfair. Not that there are nice diseases, but I mean ... in their final years to forget everyone and everything that ever meant anything to them in all of their years prior to the disease ... Sigh ... Head hung a little low thinking of the woes.

FEBRUARY 25, 2015

New clothes and a new purse always make a girl smile. She walked around telling everyone, including me, that her shirt and purse were from Dayna Steele. She didn't want to put the new shirt on first until I told her Dayna Steele bought it for her. And, Dayna Steele filled her new purse with photos, the cards you send, gum, bracelets and her last phone book she keeps. Several times she took the gum out and said, "Dayna Steele brought me this." I will try to bring her a little something from Dayna Steel for her purse each time now ... suggestions?

Lipstick.

Photos from your youth or your baby pictures.

Give her (4) five-dollar bills.

A simple strand of pearls.

FEBRUARY 28, 2015

Mom is getting increasingly agitated — hard to watch someone who was so happy and bubbly most of the time, go through this. One visitor who calms her greatly is my brother Scooter. One of the sad things about this disease is the number of friends and family who disappear as the disease gets worse. I'm lucky to have Scooter. We are lucky to have each other. The best Mom in the world raised us.

Yes, it is so true how many people disappear when something like this happens.

It is so sad when people just drop out of your life. I was reading the book "Loving Someone who has Dementia" (by Pauline Boss), as I care for my mother with Alzheimer's, and it said this happens because friends/ family don't know how to comfort you. It's easy when there is a death, the typical courtesies are extended, food is brought over, cards and calls to comfort you, but during that duration of the disease, and progression of symptoms that leave us.

The caregivers in this perpetual state of grief, grieving the loss of our living family member, others don't quite know how to comfort us, because there hasn't been an actual death. It's so true and it does feel lonely to lose others while your experience losing the ones we love, yet are only living in "their own little shells." This disease is indeed horrifying.

MARCH 2, 2015

This crazy, sweet, wonderful woman who never met a stranger and always made cookies for everyone — is a bully. Yep. Miss Fran is the bully in memory care. That's the thing about this disease, it strips you of any filters you might have had in place at some time. Mom hates old people; Mom has always disliked old people. Mom has never had kind words for people who did not age gracefully. Of course, you would have never heard her say a word. Only those closest to her — Scooter and me — knew this. As the disease progressed, the filters began to fade. Things she used to say in private, started to say in a whisper then louder and louder. Then the comments turned into actions, bumping people with her walker. Anyone in her way now gets rammed with the walker. I finally had to make the decision to approve a calming medication twice a day — for a woman who had never taken so much as an aspirin. I love her so, but that left hook of hers is amazing.

The most important thing is that she is in as much peace as you can help her to be. No one should have to live their final years being someone they would not like or respect or recognize when they were younger and healthier. My mom was terrified as she entered the later stages of this insidious disease. She knew enough to know she didn't know what was going to happen next and the fear in her eyes was the hardest thing for me to cope with. My brother and I made the hard decision to limit her meds to ones that would simply reduce her fear.

My grandmother had a bad ass left hook, which she landed square on my chin, knocked me out cold as I was giving her a bath. Funny now. Soaking wet she weighed 90 lbs.

My shy and virtuous dad began hitting on the nurses and making lewd remarks. I was stunned!!

March 7, 2015

Dr. Charles Justiz and I were married 23 years ago today. I loved the whole bride thing but we did the wedding thing our usual frugal way. The cakes and photos were gifts. The dress was borrowed. HPD gave us a police escort to the airport as a gift. The venue was a free local museum and we made a small donation, $50 I think. The hotel manager was a huge KLOL fan and discounted everything like crazy. Crash was the wedding DJ as a gift and Miss Molly and the Whips played as a gift for a small fee. We stayed with friends in Cabo San Lucas for a honeymoon and borrowed their extra dune buggy. Best of all (besides Charlie) — Mom "borrowed" huge bunches of flowers from the hotel gardens and decorated the reception with those. I keep telling you, I come by it honestly …

I love this story! I love that your Mom snitched the flowers. Lolol.

MARCH 12, 2015

The more I read and the more I learn about Mom's diagnosis, the more things I look back on and say, "Oh wow — it was happening then." I had one of those moments/memories this morning. Christi Ayo had moved back to Houston in 2007 and I was telling mom how great it was to have her close again. Christi and I were the closest of friends from about the age of 13. She was my wedding maid of honor. We are talking major history together for years. Mom smiled and commented how nice that was. About five minutes later she said, " Now remind me again who Christi is." I remembered it stopped me in my tracks but I chalked it up to old age and didn't think about it again, until this morning. I think Mom has lived with it much longer than we imagined but she was so darn organized, had such a routine and became so good at covering it up that it has only been in the latter stages that we realized something was wrong. I now continually wonder: Was she scared? Did she know? Could I have made it easier?

We learn as young children to answer questions in a way that will elicit favorable responses.

Unless you know the specific way to ask a question to someone with Alzheimer's, they will give you the 'right answer' every time.

MARCH 23, 2015

Arrived home in Houston airport about 9:30 last night. First thought for a split second was — it's probably too late to call Mom, can't wait to tell her about the Cuba trip. Those times I want to pick up the phone and call her and tell her about something the boys have done or a new pair of shoes or another exciting family adventure — then I realize I can't — not because she is gone but because she is gone in another way. Definition of a 'lump in your throat.'

There are some days, though, when there is clarity. You for a moment, think, "She is better!" But you realize it's just a gift for the moment. Lump in the throat.

That is the best thing about parents when you are an adult: Having someone to call and tell about the little things, knowing that they will care when no one else would in quite the same way. I remember feeling the same with my Dad. He was there physically, but he was already lost to me. At some point, you end up going through your grieving process before they die.

MARCH 29, 2015

There is less and less to write and observe as we enter the sixth stage of Alzheimer's — most often defined as: "Severe Cognitive decline. Memory continues to worsen, personality changes may take place and individuals need extensive help with daily activities." Visits are becoming increasingly hard on her; though happy to see us, it disrupts the routine and she gets aggressive/angry when we leave — but forgets we were there minutes later. As we left yesterday, Nick said "Mimi just doesn't seem like herself anymore." He was carefully trying to say something but was scared how to put it — so I said it. "She looks like a mean old lady." He looked relieved that I saw it, too. We are in a state of limbo — we are just waiting for the inevitable. And the often wished for at this stage.

Wow I do understand. Soon she will forget how to eat and drink. This can last a really long time, seems like forever for you. Care facilities make $ by trying to prolong life, care workers can be overtired and occasionally hit back so visits now are more safety checks and advocacy for kindness/comfort. Stop taking her out, as patients are just frightened and disoriented with any changes. Also I would stop bringing the kids, as this will be the memory of their precious grandmother, better to reinforce great memories for them and for you.

March 31, 2015

Conversation my entire life, since the day I learned to speak.
Me: I don't like Jell-O.
Mom: You don't?
Me: NO, I don't like Jell-O
Mom: Are you sure?
Me: I am very sure. I hate Jell-O.
Mom: Sure you don't want to try a taste?
Me: No.
Yesterday I prepped for a regular colonoscopy. Jell-O was my friend for a brief few hours. Don't tell Mom.

Your secret is safe with us!

Come on Everyone Loves Jell-O!!!

April 2, 2015

There is nothing like a grandmother's smile and a grandmother's hug. Oh, those are missed. Maybe not so much by the boys but by me watching Mom and the boys interact. There isn't any of that anymore. Recently out to eat, a grandmother came into the restaurant to meet her family. The two grand-kids jumped up to hug her — all three beaming. I didn't realize I missed that until I saw it. Strong emotions will overtake you when you least expect it.

It's a very slow process. Just take it one day at a time.

As a grandmother of three amazing kids this one hit me hard.

Little insights.

April 6, 2015

It's heartbreaking to look at this image — her nails aren't done, her hair is a mess and she has a black eye. She is very paranoid about people touching her so I do her nails as I can (if she lets me) and will attempt to get her hair done again this week. As for the black eye, she is at a stage where she is los-ing her balance. Like a toddler, if you take your eyes of her for a minute, she will get into some sort of trouble like forgetting to use her walker. She for-gets immediately what happened and doesn't seem to hurt. That said, she's happy or at least her current version of happy. We bring her the occasional Dr Peppers, Subway sandwiches, and dog visits. Someone commented to me privately the other day that I may be sharing too much in these posts. I have to. It is cathartic for me and all the books I have read and research I have done never prepared me for these so personal moments. Sharing with you is my anchor as I keep one foot in this other bizarre new world.

People need to know.

You're not sharing too much, Dayna. You're doing what you have to do to stay sane. If it helps you then that's all that matters.

There is nothing that can prepare anyone for this insidious disease.

I go through this same process with my Mom; it helps me more than you can ever know to read these posts.

It makes all my little shit just little shit!

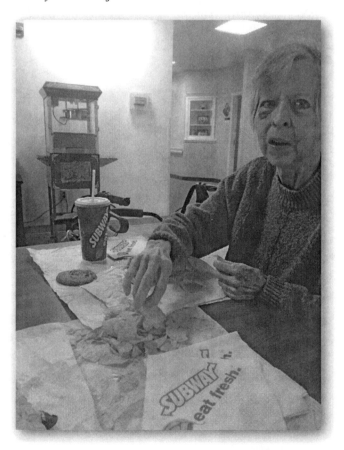

April 23, 2015

After spending the week in Austin, with an exhibit at the University of Texas, about Mom's journey with this disease, it was sweet to come back and spend some time with her. Her real exhibit has not shut down yet. She seems more frail now, a little smaller, sleeping more, less interested in whatever I bring — or me. And one new thing I really noticed. There are no books. I come from a family of readers; I'm a reader. My kids are readers. Mom was a reader. Even though she couldn't read any more, she has been hoarding books from the facility library in her room for months. We put them away and days later she has five to ten books all over her room again. Books are comforting to us. This visit, no books! Not a one. She's not interested. She has forgotten books.

Alzheimer's just sucks ... I hate it ...

My grandmother has Alzheimer's and has lost interest in a lot of things.

It always helped me to think of my mom as a simply beautiful soul in an earth suit. And the suit wore out, but her soul was strong and bright within it.

April 27, 2015

Mom has gotten to the point where she needs more care, more attention, and more compassion. Moving her to a private Alzheimer's care home that came highly recommended and is close. These moves are hard on her and hard on me — wondering if I made a wrong decision on the last place and am I making the right decision on the next place. It is also hard to get rid of more of her things with each move. The good news, she will have more purpose in her last months, doing things she wants to do like helping in the kitchen and playing with her dog in a real backyard. I find myself often telling her, "I'm doing the best I can Mom. The best I can." I don't know if she understands at all but I hope. Send her a note? She loves those and carries them around in her walker: Fran Nicholson c/o Light Heart, 910 Kingsgate, Houston, TX 77058.

It's so hard to know I vacillate between thinking she's in a good place and freaking out that they are missing things, and my siblings are NO help.

Don't question yourself or your decisions.

Forget about second-guessing — that's what we do on sports talk radio!

There is no manual.

When I was visiting my Grandmother who was in long-term care a gentleman came up to her and said, "Have you seen my wife?" My Grandma replied "No, but will I do?"

MAY 10, 2015

Happy Mother's Day! I have so many wonderful things from mom I try to remember: My ability to talk to anyone anywhere, great brownie and cookie recipes, a love of cooking for everyone, too many animals, travel lust, and a super charged metabolism. This morning my mother will wake up and not remember me. Sometime in the morning she will remember me. She'll remember the 30-year old me that is still on the radio. And, then she'll get mad at me, because the 30-year old me is not there. When I come to visit, she will smile to greet a visitor but then get a frantic look on her face at the same time. The look that says get me out of here, I need to find the 30-year old Dayna. Is your Mom still around? Hug, love, visit, call — something. And do it every day not just Mother's Day. It is terribly sad when you can't. Or she can't.

This is a wonderful tribute.

Courage!

May 13, 2015

Wish I had more dark humor for you but I think we may have progressed beyond that now. There wasn't a whole lot of recognition the first part of my last visit. And, Mom spent a good part of our Mother's Day visit hitting me. That's a new one. She has hit others and still hits her image in mirrors and reflections. The caregivers have told me this is a phase some patients go through, that she will come out of it eventually — then becoming more catatonic, even less awareness or understanding. Not sure which is worse. Here is a good, short piece on Alzheimer's rage: http:/www.webmd.com/alzheimers-agression

> *Thank you for sharing so honestly. It really helps others to deal with their feelings … just knowing other people understand what they are going through.*

> *I believe they are in there so keep beaming!!*

May 17, 2015

There is so very little that makes her smile and seem in the least bit happy these days. One is her dog and the other is true for just about any woman of any age — just getting her nails and hair done. Enough said.

> *Alzheimer's is just a pendulum of so many stages, so many emotions so much pain for those in it and those out of it.*

MAY 22, 2015

Just when you think there is no humor to be found, I laughed yesterday. I went to see her right before dinner. She asks over and over again if I am taking her to my house. She shows no interest in anything but I brought her my new book. She thumbed through the pages three times and would not put it down. It made me feel good. Then dinner was served and all bets were off. We may be tiny but boy do we love to eat. Yep, another thing I come by honestly — get out of the way, there's food! I was able to leave without any problem. I chuckled all the way to the car. It was a good visit. It was a good day.

Every day is a new day. Enjoy each and every one, even though it's painful at times.

Cherish the good days.

MAY 24, 2015

Mom is losing the ability to speak, to say very much. She is very hard to understand when she does talk but I know what she is saying — it is some form of "are you taking me to your house?" Over and over again. I had one of those weird moments of clarity again a few days ago. In the middle of asking me this over and over, she paused, looked off for a moment, then visibly sat up straight, looked me squarely in the eye and in her old, strong voice said, " I don't even remember what your kitchen looks like." She looked off into space again and went right back into the weak, repeated question and frail body. Sometimes these moments of clarity are nice, other times they are just spooky. Some people never get any; some may get one or two. We've had several. And for the record, I don't know what my kitchen looks like either.

Those moments of clarity with my mother would leave me emotionally drained.

Played dementia version of "Who's on First?" with my mother-in law today. She brought up a party. I didn't know of a party. I asked her about the party. She said, "What party?" You're in my thoughts and prayers.

My wife's great aunt lives with us in Ecuador, and is in the advanced stage. She often sits in the living room with a view of the river, while I take calls in my home office. She rarely talks now, and always looks at me trying to figure out who is this gringo sitting at the table. Last week she was helped into her chair for breakfast, then she lifted her head, beamed a smile, and said "Good morning! How is everyone doing today?" Never mind that she doesn't, or didn't, know a word of English.

I truly never grasped that I truly never grasped what "The Long Goodbye" meant until you started these updates. You have taught us so much.

MAY 27, 2015

This is hard. Fucking hard. Hit an emotional wall today. Think the floods and the deaths and despair of strangers opened up suppressed emotions. Weepy mess. Fuck.

Sometimes we need to be emotional instead of keeping it all bottled inside and when we need to be strong, we are strong! There is no instructional book on how to take care of our parents with Alzheimer's but we do what we can with what is in our hearts, don't worry about the future, forget the past, and live for this moment!

Cry, sometimes it is the best medicine.

There is tremendous strength in allowing yourself to fully feel these emotions.

Yeah. Fuck. Fuckitall!!

Dayna sometimes FUCK is the only word that describes it all!! Hang tough.

Dayna note: Finding the perfect word is nirvana for a writer. For those who were or are offended, I'm sorry, fuck is the most perfect word ever invented for some situations.

MAY 28, 2015

I'm better today — thanks to you. Your messages of concern and support have been tremendous and much appreciated. Please know that as weepy as I was yesterday, Mom actually had one of her best days we've seen in a long time. She has always been creative, was always an artist. Look at this smile. I spent 30 minutes helping my mother color. Fifty years ago, she did the same for me. This disease just gets stranger and more surreal each day …

Brilliant keeping her creative side engaged.

Wow that's the reality of it right there.

The last time my dad told me he loved me was when he was finishing a foam puzzle for a 2 to 3 year old with my help. There is real beauty and grace in meeting them "where they are." Your posts are helping me remember this.

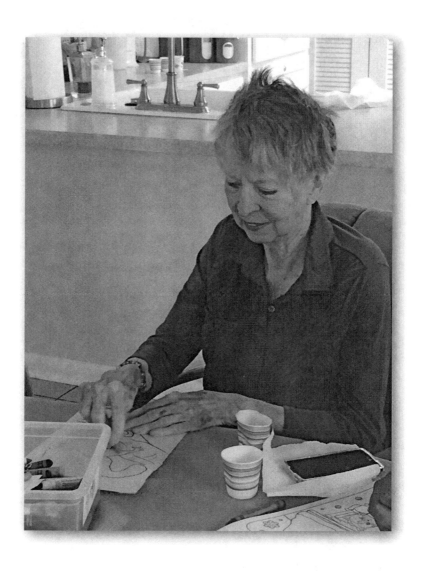

JUNE 2, 2015

You learn all sorts of tricks. Coloring keeps her still. Live entertainers keep her attention, and recorded music does not! She doesn't sit for TV or iPads ... unless I'm on one. She will sit for a bit and smile if her dog is in her lap. And, the new one, you can get her hair done without her hitting the stylist if candy is involved.

Great information. I need to try candy. Some for Mom and some for me!

What a curse Alzheimer's is ... we dealt with it like so many other families ... it's a tough one when they are there in body but not in mind.

JUNE 4, 2015

Now that she can barely speak, I started thinking of some of the things she always said:
-Do you want some Jell-O?
-Don't throw that out, put it in the freezer.
-Don't shuffle your feet.
-Where are the good scissors?
I miss these things now but they used to drive me crazy. You? What's your favorite Mom phrase?

In or out! We're not trying to air condition the outside!

Boy you need that like you need a hole in your head!

If everybody jumped in the lake, would you do it, too?

Pretty is as pretty does.

Where are the good scissors?

Don't make that face. It might stay that way.

Because I said so!

If you're bored start cleaning.

Don't forget to call me when you get there.

Jesus, Mary, and Joseph. I didn't know it was profane; I thought it was just an exclamation she used instead of the cussing. So I said it at school at a very young age and got into a heap of trouble. Somehow, I still say it sometimes, and I never see it coming. Oh Mom.

Don't make me come in there.

If I wanted the world to know I would have told them.

Uglier than homemade soap.

If you lay down with dogs, you'll get up with fleas.

Put that book down and turn off the light.

There's a difference between being the boss and being bossy.

The road to hell is paved with good intentions.

Scooter Nicholson (Dayna's brother, Fran's son):
The birds will eat it.
Save that for the ducks
Who left the gate open?
What do you mean you don't like liver?
I love you a bushel and a peck and a hug around your neck.
And, I just knew when she yelled out Scooter Bill Nicholson ... I was in trouble!! And I never touched the good scissors!

Dayna note: This is one of my favorite posts. There were literally hundreds of responses, way too many to put here. This one post may be a book all on its own some day.

June 16, 2015

She's forgetting people quickly (or it seems quickly now). She's very wary of Son 3.0 and doesn't know who Son 1.0 is. But she still loves her a good-looking man.

She is a big flirt! LOL!

The woman isn't stupid.

June 21, 2015

There is the occasional strange moment of clarity. I've experienced it a couple of times. My aunt and uncle saw one the other day. It is as if she is back for a few seconds, then returns to her current advanced state in this disease. What worries me? In those few seconds is she scared?

I would imagine that those are a welcomed time of clarity and control and that other times are scary ... much like being a toddler, absent of vocabulary on the playground with older children.

I think they are a brief respite and blessing for all involved.

JUNE 29, 2015

I've been gone for two weeks and need to see Mom. I said need, not want. That's one of the feelings I now hate about this disease. I find an excuse not to go. Doctors and friends say she has no concept of time and that I may be disrupting her routine when I do go. I could go every day and she would say I never visit. I could go twice a month and she might think I was there all the time. The visits aren't for her; they are for me, to make it feel like I'm doing the right thing. That I'm a good daughter. That I'm taking care of her. It's such an unpleasant visit sometimes — she's mad, hates old people (always has) and may hit me. She glares at Nick. She looks so old and not herself. She isn't herself. And I don't want to go ...

You are showing your children how to take care of a parent when they can no longer take care of themselves. Be warned, your children are watching.

All of our parents are nearing the end of the road. Some may be facing more potholes than others, but for none it's not an easy goodbye. We were no cakewalk as toddlers, I bet. Life's cycle of love!

It's a tough dance. Hang in there.

I think it was Mother Teresa who said do good anyway ...

JUNE 30, 2015

Spent time with Mom last night. (Thanks for all your kind words yester-day.) I took her a Diet Dr Pepper, her favorite. She drank a bit then gave up. Noticed she is having a hard time swallowing. I have done enough reading to know what that means ....

Late or end stage Alzheimer's or other dementia usually requires intensive care. Get insight on what to expect, the role of the caregiver etc.

Swallowing isn't automatic. It can be forgotten like so many other things Alzheimer's takes away. Hopefully staff is monitoring this.

July 7, 2015

Thanks for all the suggestions of ways to entertain mom and make her happy. Colors and coloring sheets are nice, they keep her busy but must be very, very simple, like for a toddler. She hates headphones so personal music players are out. A staff member sings hymns to her, and she likes that. Music playing in the background sounds like noise to most Alzheimer's patients. The simple truth is that we have finally come to grips with the fact that nothing will make her happy. If it does, it is only for a few brief moments and she goes back to being mad and irritated, trying to hit us or other residents. That's a hard one to grasp or even type but it is true. I hear it all the time — people who were mean and nasty pre-disease are now the happiest, most pleasant people to be around. Or the opposite; such as in our case. It does not stop us from trying. Thanks to Ames Arlan, CEO of Arlan's Markets. I told him she used to shell purple hull peas for hours (I hated those damn peas). He delivered a box full of bags of peas to be shelled along with flowers — making me cry in the grocery store. She sat for an hour with me alternating between helping, eating the raw peas, and throwing them at me. But it was a good hour with my mommy …

Pop beads are fun. Target has a big jar. My young grandkids love them.

Choose to see these times as a sign of your ability for compassion. The moments of her difficulties with you are so far in the past you were too young to remember. She will be your most cherished memory down the road. Even today she still teaches you, though in a far different way.

We brought my Mom a bag of cracked pecans. She knew exactly what to do with them. And we all enjoyed eating the pecans of course!

My grandma was the sweetest person in the world and when she cursed like a sailor, I had to pick my mouth up off the ground, walk out of the room, regroup and back into the tranches! I will never forget that first time! Bless you, your mom and your family!

JULY 13, 2015

I have been on the road for two weeks. I got a call from Mom's care-giver. "It's her birthday tomorrow. What do you have planned?" I was horrified that I could have forgotten my own Mother's birthday. Have I written her off that easily already? Tears flowed as I cried on a friend's shoulder. How could I forget something so iconic as 9/11, Mom's birth date?"
Friend: It's July 11th.
Me: Oh. Then why the hell did this floor me and confuse me so badly.
Friend: This disease comes with an unbelievable amount of guilt for family members. You are probably already feeling awful for being gone for two weeks. Anything could have set you off. This was it.
Me: Open another bottle of wine.

I guess every day is a special day.

You are so focused day to day on her well-being, and what this devastating disease is robbing her (and all of you) of that the dates really don't come in to play, only the days and the moments.

JULY 14, 2015

Leaving Cheap Trick's studio last night in Nashville. In the car, leaving the driveway, a friend's son mentions that their producer worked with Glen Campbell on his Alzheimer's song. I made Wonder Husband stop the car and went running back to hug Julian Raymond, co-writer and producer of Glen Campbell's "I'm Not Gonna Miss You" — I cried and told him how much it meant to me. It is a song that captures the disease. Julian said Glen no longer knows anyone but laughs, smiles and hugs everyone. So wish that was Mom! Thanks Julian.

> *Love this song so much. My husband of 52 years passed away on June 14. Your updates always made me feel better.*

> *The disease terrorizes me.*

> *That incredible song and the documentary brought me to my knees. I see it getting closer and I can't stop it.*

I'M NOT GONNA MISS YOU
by Glen Campbell and Julian Raymond

I'm still here, but yet I'm gone
I don't play guitar or sing my songs
They never defined who I am
The man that loves you 'til the end
You're the last person I will love
You're the last face I will recall
And best of all,

I'm not gonna miss you
Not gonna miss you

I'm never gonna hold you like I did
Or say I love you to the kids
You're never gonna see it in my eyes
It's not gonna hurt me when you cry
I'm never gonna know what you go through
All the things I say or do
All the hurt and all the pain
One thing selfishly remains

I'm not gonna miss you
I'm not gonna miss you

*Special thanks to the Campbell family and Julian Raymond
for permission to reprint these lyrics*

July 20, 2015

We are on another family flying adventure this week. Many say — oh I wish I could just take off and go places. You can. And should. I took Mom to London and Hawaii. We had plans to go to Las Vegas on 9/11. Then Dad had a stroke and we kept putting it off. When she could finally travel with me again — she couldn't. I think about that on each and every adventure — whether it is on a beach in Italy or a trip to the local farmers market in Seabrook. There is something I do everyday that makes me think Mom would have loved this. Don't wait. Have adventures now with the ones you love. Adventure is to be found everywhere. YOU create the adventure. Mom would have loved that.

OMG! So very true!

JULY 24, 2015

Saw Mom for the first time in almost three weeks, been traveling. That's one of the hard things, just moving on and living your life with the ones who are still here and need you the most — yourself, your partner, your kids — in that order. She had more mail; thanks Heather and Suzy. That keeps her occupied. I brought Dr Pepper and Chick-fil-A (sometimes you have to suppress your politics and beliefs for the good of others.) She's starting to shake a lot — ala Parkinson's. At this point, I won't put her through any testing or medication unless she is in pain. I can't believe this just goes on and on. And on and on and on! *Bonus: I have no idea whose clothes she is wearing. Get used to that in any facility — big or small — it just all gets mixed up.

Wow, this is bringing back all kinds of wounds I didn't know I had.

I showed up to check on my grandmother one Sat. morning, to my shock she had the biggest set of false teeth in her mouth that she had grabbed from some poor man's room. We never did find her teeth. It was the funniest sight.

An RN, aka an angel, once told me: "You're in the middle of your life; she's at the end of hers." It was some of the best advice she could give.

AUGUST 4, 2015

Move number six took place yesterday. Another Light Heart facility to see if it makes her less agitated*. They asked me to stay away and let them handle it, so no "transference" would take place — meaning she would be mad at me about the move and the old people. This way, they are the bad guys and I can sweep in today with a Diet Dr Pepper and her dog and be a hero, telling her how much I love her new place. At first I was so relieved when they asked me not to come. Then, I felt tremendously guilty for being so happy to stay away. Then, sad that I wasn't there to move her, wasn't needed this time. And then, resigned to knowing this really was the right way to handle it. Caregivers promised her a milkshake for the short journey. She can be bought. One of the residents looked a little like my late Dad. Mom was pretty agitated with the real Dad his last few years. I think in her own mind she was telling this resident what to do (even though she is non-verbal) and she was constantly clapping her hands at him and hitting him when she passed him because he wasn't minding her. Yes, it is a bizarre journey we are on ...

The hardest journey ...

Alzheimer's is a disease that many people are not familiar with and this gives us all an idea of what is expected and how it can be handled. Thank you so much!

A reminder that we're not alone in the trials and tribulations of those caring for loved ones with Alzheimer's.

August 5, 2015

Thanks for the overwhelming response to yesterday's tip. In answer to several questions:
Yes, I'm fine. These posts are very cathartic for me and writing them helps like you would never imagine. And to the stranger, who attacked me for posting these updates, just know my Mom loved being the center of attention — especially if she was helping people.
And yes, this is turning into a book.

Pooh on people who don't get it ... it is cathartic. It also lets others who are in your shoes know they are not alone: smile emoticon.

It was always helpful for me to read blogs from others going through what I was. Keep writing. For those of us that are in the same situation, it helps to hear your experiences. It lets us know that we are not alone and we can possibly share valuable information and offer support.

I'm glad I didn't see the post. What a dumbass. I would have been DELIGHTED to go pregnant on them!

August 10, 2015

Mom is getting settled in her new place. We've done six moves so far. The first few we worked so hard to move her things and decorate, things that would make her feel comfortable and at home. With each subsequent move, we took fewer and fewer things. It's been so strange to watch an entire life-time of memories dwindle over the past two years into one box now. And, I think these things are more for us than her. Not sure she has any idea who most of the people in the pictures are anymore. The things are a physical representation of what her brain is doing with memories. One box.

This is the definition of a poignant moment. My heart goes out to you and your family. The way you deal with this and share it, including the humor you find, must be a big help to others going through the same journey. Bless you.

The old saying, "You can't take it with you," should be how anyone one on the backside of life should think about belongings. Don't leave your kids with your crap.

My grandma had really bad paranoia as well. She would take all of the stuff off of the walls because she thought the workers would try to steal them. Especially pictures. My grandma was always a picture person. I made her a scrapbook that she would hide under her mattress. She looked at it often, even when she didn't know the people anymore.

I have been through this "Ground Hog Days" saga too many times!

AUGUST 16, 2015

My friend asked me the other day if Mom ever seems scared. I ask myself that all the time. She was a pretty sharp woman and had to have known something was happening. If she ever went to a doctor for a diagnosis, she didn't tell us. I wonder if she was terrified it was happening then, she had to have known. I so wish I had known and could have comforted her. We are in the final stages of Alzheimer's now — where nothing is black and white. Is she scared? Yes. Of what? No one will ever know. Are we strangers? Do our voices hurt her ears? Do we look like monsters? Does she know she's supposed to know us and doesn't and that's frightening? Yes, she looks scared to me. And, I try everything to make it better not knowing what she is scared of or having any idea what demons we are fighting ...

My father was frightened almost every minute he was awake after his stroke, which caused his dementia! That was the hardest thing to deal with!

That fear and anxiety and not being able to soothe it is the worst part of dementia and Alzheimer's to me.

Way back in the seventies we were taught that in Alzheimer's there is no awareness of memory loss. We were taught a lot of things which I do not believe or have since been disproven. Yes, I think most people recognize they are having more trouble. Another thing is lack of ability to complain if there is pain somewhere: dental, bladder, headache, etc. so those things make people angrier, and behavioral symptoms are the symptom (like a newborn crying, gotta figure it out).

AUGUST 19, 2015

When I moved mom from a facility to a private home, I took the last of all of her apartment-type things and threw them in my closet. I just could not go through and discard things one more time. Usually when someone dies, you go through things once and do what you have to do with everything and be done with it. This has been a two- and a half-year process, getting rid of a few more things each move (six now as the disease progresses). I was beaten down. Finally went through things this past weekend to sort into save for sons and nieces, give to brother, hold on to for my memories, send to Goodwill, etc. One thing left to go through. Can't do it just yet. Her last Dayna Steele scrapbook. She was my biggest fan ...

You're doing great — took me 10 years to go through the last of my mom's boxes.

Remember to take photos of things before you discard them or give them away if they are meaningful to you, that way you can still see them if you feel like reminiscing.

Ok she can be first but I'm your second biggest fan!!!

AUGUST 26, 2015

Every time the phone rings and it's a number I don't recognize or it's mom's caregivers, I hope it's "the call." At the same time, I hope it's not "the call." I dread, "the call" but want "the call" at the same time. When you find out it's not "the call," it's a mixed bag of feelings including relief and disappointment. You know "the call" is coming, just not when. Then I go to visit her and think, "the call" can wait for now.

This part of life needs to be discussed.

Roller coaster of emotions.

No way I can click "like" on this ... profound.

She looks like she's waiting for the call as well.

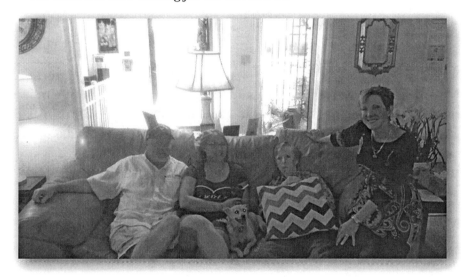

September 1, 2015

She hits everyone and everything, even her beloved dog Sandy. We don't take Sandy anymore because the dog is now scared of Mom. Since Mom hits Sandy, we don't really think it is anger or frustration — we're just not sure what it is. And there is no easy explanation for why an Alzheimer's patient does anything. Our wonderful neighbor Cheryl still drops by with her trained therapy dog Mija. Mom hits both and they both keep smiling. A lucky neighbor I am to have them.

My mom, when I asked her to stand up, would often let her legs go limp. Or I would ask her to take a step forward and she'd step back. Connections are switched in the brain.

Most people don't realize that the stress on the caregiver is often many times greater than the stress felt by the patient!

The internal controls over behaviors and words are gone. It is so hurtful for those of us who are left. I am thankful my dad never got physically mean, he would just say things (that were true to him) but hurtful.

SEPTEMBER 4, 2015

I was looking back this past week and found myself so sad that there is no more dark humor, only sadness, and the wait. Or so I thought. Brought Mom a Chick-fil-A kid's meal (her favorite for years). Toy inside? A book of Brain Games! Come on — ya gotta laugh!

Oh boy!

Gotta love it, never give up

I laughed. Love you!

SEPTEMBER 8, 2015

Radio legend Scott Sparks touched my heart the other day by asking this question: what still brings your Mom joy? Dr Pepper. That's about it. So we bring one every visit. Do you have a question? About her, how I cope, the disease, your own challenges caring for a loved one with Alzheimer's? Ask here and I'll do my best to answer all.

You have taught me to treasure each moment with mine, to catalog our old stories and memories, and to laugh/cry/listen/gossip/support/cherish/love with all my might. I have had some of the most profound and life-changing discussions and experiences with my immediate family lately and I owe a great debt to you. Thank you for taking us along on your journey.

Thank you for your willingness to share this personal journey. We are in the beginning stages with our mom as she was diagnosed two years ago.

I cry all the way to visit my mom, compose myself before entering the facility with a put-on happy face, only to cry the entire journey back home. I don't live close by, and she still doesn't understand that I can't be there in 5 minutes. And 5 minutes seems like 30 to her.

Do you ever want to give up? Like get so discouraged that you never want to go back visit?

Dayna note: Almost daily. I procrastinate when it comes to seeing her, I just don't want to go. And I so want this over. We are better to our animals than we are our old and dying. Then I remember she probably got tired of me at times and still took care of me.

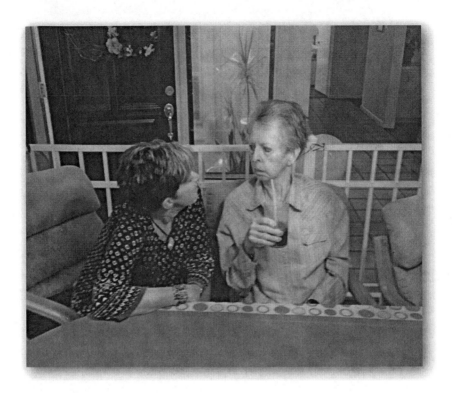

SEPTEMBER 11, 2015

Miss Fran is 86 today. Does she know what a birthday is? I don't think so. Is the attention good? Or is it too much and we're just doing it for ourselves? She got a Dr Pepper. Nothing else, she throws everything else. Music, stuffed animals, puzzles, coloring books — thanks for all the suggestions — but no. They don't work. She seemed to watch the US Tennis Open this week. Not sure she can see it but boy she knows the sound of a good serve after all her years of A-team tennis. Here's a card I found for her years ago. Going through her things she had saved it. Some card I found at an airport somewhere in the world — it is NOT her — but oh my it looks just like her. Made us both crack up. Still does for one of us.

Happy birthday, Flo. I cherish the nights spent at your table scarfing down chicken spaghetti and buying gold jewelry. That pile of gold was a good investment. I miss you.

My mom was taking a walk last week and fell, broke a bone in her hand and knocked out 3 teeth, lots of bruises and skin tears. I talked to her yesterday, she couldn't remember my name.

My mom is 86 also and currently in a rehab facility. She fell after a doctor's appointment as we were leaving. Reading your posts has helped me come to grips with the thought she may never be right again.

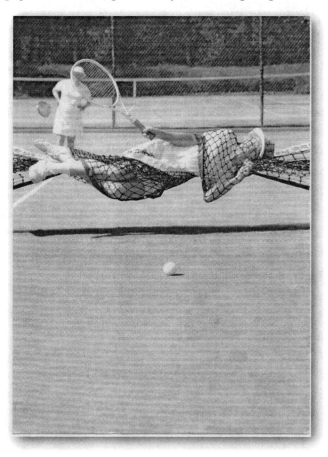

September 14, 2015

The Facebook flashbacks are taking me by surprise. Takes breath away. Unexpected tears. Large wine.

I know what you mean — I'll have vodka, thank you.

She would smile again if she could. Just having your love keeps her smiling on the inside when she can't show emotion on outside.

September 21, 2015

The thing that makes me the saddest right now is that there is nothing I can do to make my mom happy, even the Dr Pepper doesn't do what I am looking for. Beth Middleton suggested I play one of my old radio recordings for Mom. Oh my. Oh my. She froze like an unruly kid hearing their mom's voice. Then relaxed, put her head down on my phone, closed her eyes, the stress in her face disappeared and she almost smiled. I only have two saved shows. She listened and never moved. Looking at me with almost begging eyes for more when it ended. She hated coming back to her reality. She wanted more. I will find her more. Did you ever record my radio show? Still have a cassette tucked away in a drawer somewhere? I need it, will pay for the postage, will pick it up, will copy it, and return it. My biggest fan needs it.

This made me smile and my eyes leak. So happy you found something that made her heart smile ... and yours too.

It's very hard to make someone happy. Especially hard when that person has lost the cognizant idea of what it means to be happy.

The mother's voice calms the child in the womb; the child's voice calms the mother in the shell.

You are locked in her memory and always there with her.

SEPTEMBER 23, 2015

Lovely pink shirt today. It's not hers. Nor are the pants. That's one thing you have to get used to in care facilities. She was such a put together woman. Always dressed well, accessorized, color coordinated, etc. Now there is no jewelry (she may eat or throw it) and the clothes are rarely hers. Keeping up with clothes are the least of the worries — for her, family, or hired caregivers — you have to let go of that one. She hit me most of the visit. So I held her hand and told her I loved her. They are recommending we start hospice in the next week or so. Sorry to blurt that out. I'm having wine with my tears.

Those were the toughest words we had to hear with my mom. Be there for her just like you are doing now.

My mother started hospice care in February and it actually was a huge relief. The nurses and other staff are so wonderful in their care of the patient - and the family.

The clothes thing used to drive my aunts crazy at the facility my grandma was in. They finally had to embrace it as well.

This reminds me of when I went to visit Mom and noticed how much weight she had lost because her glasses were even way too big now. Carolyn looked at her and then said "Well hell ... they're not her's!" We laughed so hard!

Thank you for sharing the part about wearing other people's clothes. It's the one thing that gives me a slight chuckle when I visit my mom. I joke with her and ask her if she went shopping without telling anyone. Hell, my grandmother was buried in someone else's dress.

September 30, 2015

Mom would so embarrass me wherever we went: Do you know Dayna Steele? Did you ever listen to Dayna Steele? Do you ever read any of Dayna Steele's books? Well, this is Dayna Steele! Mom! After a long meeting with lots of tears (mine) yesterday, the decision was made to put Mom in hospice today. Here's how the Physician's Assistant's phone call with the hospice provider went:

PA: I need to recommend a patient for hospice.

Nurse: Is this in the Clear Lake area?

PA: Yes.

Nurse: Is the patient female?

PA: Uh, yes.

Nurse: Is her daughter kind of famous?

PA: (wide-eyed) Yes ...

Nurse: Is the daughter's name Dayna?

PA: Yes. How do you know this?

Nurse: Oh wow — I have followed this story on Facebook. I am so glad you called me. We will be there tomorrow to help Dayna and her Mom.

I have always appreciated my Steeleworker network. Today, I am blown away by you. I swear Mom was trying to smile when I left ... she will be my #1 Steeleworker to the very end.

It takes a village ...

Hospice workers are angels. She will be in good hands.

What a blessing, a network is always so worthwhile when they have your best interest and sounds like this group does.

Just when you think this story can't get any more heart wrenching ...

I miss your Mom already.

It's been an honor to be allowed to share this journey with you.

October 4, 2015

Mom has never been sick, only been in a hospital twice to have children, no broken bones, drank tons of water, never took prescription drugs, ate well, exercised, was always thin, did crossword puzzles all the time, no stress, was happy, worked at a creative job — all the things you are supposed to do to stave off this disease. So we were blindsided by Alzheimer's — as most are. We never discussed assisted living or memory care. Did not think we would need it. She had everything else written down and ready to go, even her obits are pre-written for us. Have the conversation today with your loved ones — no matter what age you are. Make your desires very clear. Now. Today. Have the talk. Write it all down. Make sure it is somewhere easily found. By the way, look at the date on this. We think she knew something was up this early and hid it for that long.

Amazingly mind blowing. Thanks for sharing. Definitely something to think about.

We just had our sit down meeting with our mom and it was emotional but mom has everything she wants in order and now we know as her kids that we're going to be able to respect her wishes as she desires when that time comes. This is a must for everyone having elderly parents to have "that talk" and discuss and sort things out and it accomplishes so much for when that time does come that none of us will ever be ready for. Good post.

You have no idea how many people are not prepared. Sadly, most will not take the time to take care of this.

You encourage all of us how important these talks are with our aging parents.

A Personal Message

Dearest ___ Dayna + Scooter ___.

In trying to ease the burden for you and the rest of my survivors, I have taken the time to write down my thoughts and desires. In so doing, I am attempting to make this most painful, stressful and confusing time just a bit easier to cope with.

I have tried to do as much as I could. Please accept my apologies for anything I may have overlooked.

It is with my deepest love, concern and respect for all of you that I have recorded my plans and final wishes.

Signed: ___ Mom ___

Date: ___ 7/1/09 ___

OCTOBER 7, 2015

As we near the end, I still try to pinpoint when this started and what I missed all those years. You want to think you could have made a difference and that's the real sucky thing about this disease. It still would not have mattered but we could have at least been more prepared if we had known.

She couldn't understand my Dad's dementia, she could never grasp email or the web, there were notes everywhere on everything, she sent a $5,000 bracelet to the wrong person (who fortunately sent it back), she was losing money, she started getting lost, she was frantic at dinner and couldn't sit and follow the conversations, she told Son 2.0 she didn't understand what the signs on the freeway meant anymore — and the list goes on.

We all need more awareness of this illness.

Yes, it's much more, and different than simple forgetfulness in the lead in. Frequent falls. Inexplicable panics, anxieties, demand. Unexplainable swings in mood — exuberant, fearful. Unable to comprehend money amounts or material values (someone with no money shopping for multi-million dollar homes).

I would look back on my dad's life and the things he did. As I did that, I would realize some of his actions were too out of character, and I would have an "ah ha" moment. You will find yourself doing this too — even more than you are doing now. He was so good at hiding his disease. Looking back, I know he wasn't able to really follow conversations, but he had the coping mechanisms to appear to be attending totally to what was being said. He used to love to read the daily newspaper, and I now realize that he stopped reading it quite a while before we all became aware of the disease. But he continued to take the paper — it would just pile up unread.

October 12, 2015

At Houston Methodist Hospital had a Lunch & Learn last week with their leading Alzheimer's researchers.
Fascinating and frightening.

The disease is on the rise, fast.

More early onset showing up.

2 times more likely to get than breast cancer.

Only a fraction of funding goes to Alzheimer's.

May be related in some way to autism.

They are working on a vaccine.

Get better sleep. Now.

Take B6, B12 and Folate — but be careful — too much can hurt your kidneys.

The disease may be starting in our 30's.

And the kicker, wait for it. …

… with Mom having Alzheimer's, I am 4 times more likely to get it. Great.

Well, shit fire and save matches.

How come we didn't hear much about Alzheimer's growing up? Was it called something different?

Knowledge is powerful.

October 14, 2015

A rough, rough week. Went by Monday afternoon and Mom got very violent with me — scratching, pulling hair, hitting. She seems so frail yet can hit as hard as any fighter. Cried hard all the way home. Wonder Husband, friends, brother talked me down — telling me not to take it personally. She's frightened and lost. She doesn't really know who I am or what is going on, she just knows she doesn't like it. And she doesn't want us in her space. So hard because I just want to hug her and hang on.

Your normal Mother would never ever hurt you.

I think this an intellectual challenge for you as much as an emotional one.

You KNOW it is the disease, but yet, you want your MOM.

It's odd how she recognizes your radio airchecks yet can't recognize you in person.

I had put my grandmother in the tub in about 2 inches of water, gave her a bath, drain the water, dried her off, kneeling I scoop her up and just as I got her to the top of the tub she took a swing and knock me out cold ... for a few seconds. I dropped her, cracked my head open on the sink, had to call ambulance for my self. Lol I never did that again. But it broke my heart, the doctor said they have double the strength they had in their younger years. They are scared and don't know it. Moments of reality frighten them. They lash out in a desperate, frightened internal child way. Their filters no longer contain what they held in their whole life.

October 16, 2015

I literally could not bring myself to type this the last couple of days. However, you have stayed with me through this since the beginning and I need you with me to the end. Mom stopped eating or drinking three days ago. She is very frail. No violence today, too weak. She alternates holding my hand and pushing me away. I alternate fine and sobbing.

Time for good byes.

My physician wife says this is the hard part for the caregivers. As I'm sure you already know, your mom's body is signaling it's time.

We're with you to the end and beyond. When my dad was dying the doctors were still doing swallowing tests etc. He was still lucid and said, "I'm ready to die, why do I have to go through this?" I told him we needed to be sure this wasn't something he'd recover from, but that if this last test was unsuccessful we would let him go if that's what he wanted. He said, "You're a wonderful daughter." I'm certain that is what your mother would say to you if she could.

You have changed my life and so many others; I'm sure, by sharing this journey. Following you has made me become more patient and aware of what my own aging parents may be going through.

The circle of life ...

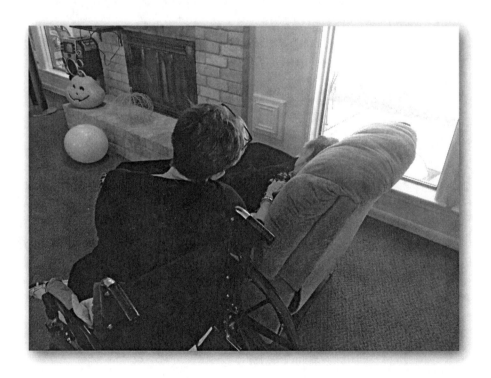

OCTOBER 17, 2015

September 11, 1929 - October 17, 2015
She lived that dash very well.

My heart is broken.

This has educated us, humanized us, and inspired us all to be better children to our aging parents.

I have been forever touched by this journey.

Thank you for sharing your mother.

Go grab some wine...

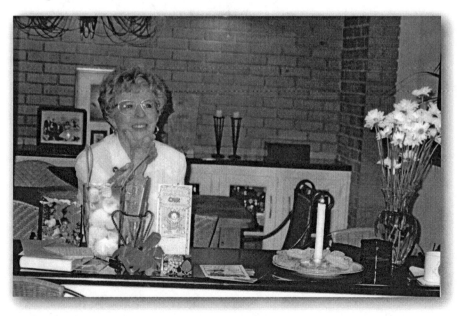

My father started growing very quiet as Alzheimer's started claiming more of him. The early stages of Alzheimer's are the hardest because that person is aware that they're losing awareness. And I think that that's why my father started growing more and more quiet. I think he felt, 'I don't want to say something wrong.' That's my sense of it.
- Patti Davis, daughter of US President Ronald Reagan

RESOURCES

THE NEUROLOGIST: DR. WILLIAM JUSTIZ

ALZHEIMER'S IS ONE of the most devastating diseases that confront the elderly today. To make matters worse, the number of people suffering from this disease is increasing since our population is living longer. Statistics on this disease are staggering. If you live to the age of 85, your chances are between 40 and 50 percent of having this disease. As this disease has no cure, it is progressive and ultimately fatal.

The worst part of Alzheimer's is that the patient loses their memories and their sense of self. Anyone afflicted will eventually forget everything if they live long enough. They will forget where they live or how to drive a car. They will forget their spouse and their children. If they live long enough, they will forget how to speak and how to walk. For this reason, the interaction between the physician and family members is important in the management of this disease. It needs to be a team approach. Families must come in with sharp ears and pencil and paper. They must come prepared with questions regarding topics they do not fully comprehend and be prepared to speak with the physician on these topics. They must listen to what the physician has to say. The physician must reciprocate and listen to the family's concerns and questions. The physician must understand that many times he/she must assume the role of psychologist and just let the family vent their anger and pain so the family can proceed through one of the most difficult times in their lives. At other times, the physician must be a cheerleader and point out the excellent work the family is doing under very psychologically and financially stressful circumstances.

When a patient comes into a neurologist's office for the first time regarding this disease, it is essential that the family members or caregiver come in with them. Even in the earliest stages of this disease the patient may not understand that they have an issue. They are either in denial, or the disease has affected the part of the brain that allows them to understand that there is truly a problem. Because of this, many first-time patients are reluctant to be in a neurologist's office and are resistant to cooperate with the physical examination. A seasoned neurologist may take this as a sign that there may be something going on.

The first visit with the patient is mostly an information-gathering visit where the neurologist is trying to understand where the patient was five years ago and where they are now. The doctor is trying to understand if there has been a change in the patient's situation. The family is critical to this stage in the process. Without the family's input, the patient may maintain enough ability to deflect any inquiry and lead the doctor to believe there is nothing abnormal ongoing with their memory. As a team, the family and the neurologist can better try to define the problems and delineate their severity.

To make the diagnosis of Alzheimer's disease, a doctor examines the patient for memory loss, which is progressive in nature. Neurologists look for signs of possible executive malfunction (cognitive abilities that control and regulate other abilities and behaviors that are necessary for goal-directed behavior), agnosia (the inability to recognize and identify objects or persons), apraxia (difficulty or impossibility in making certain motor movements, even though muscles are normal), or aphasia (loss of ability to understand or express speech). Also, during initial visits, neurologists are interested in knowing if the patient has had a history of severe head trauma, alcohol abuse, brain surgery, meningitis or even psychiatric illness as these things may affect memory in the long haul. The alcohol history is an important one as heavy alcohol intake in midlife can have an impact later. Sometimes, this is where a patient can lead a doctor down the wrong path. Most people underestimate the amount of alcohol they consume. It helps having the family serve as independent observers who can confirm the estimates of alcohol consumption. In addition to the historical fact finding on the first visit, doctors are also interested in physically examining the patient to see if there is malfunction of the nervous system that might explain their memory loss. For example, if there is weakness or numbness on one side of the body, this may suggest something wrong with the opposite hemisphere of the brain. This may suggest a stroke, tumor, or other problems. Typically, by the end of the first visit, the physician has a fairly good idea of whether or not the patient truly has a chance of having this disease. Despite the suspicion, it always helps to do further testing to eliminate uncertainties and rule out diseases that mimic Alzheimer's.

At this point, a physician will typically recommend the patient have an MRI scan of the brain performed. Typically, blood work is recommended and the patient undergoes neuropsychological testing. The Neuropsychological Battery is a series of tests putting a patient's memory through its paces, usually performed by a psychologist. In this way, neurologists can define what parts of the memory are functioning and which parts of the memory are malfunctioning. This allows them to pick up subtle deficits in memory that may not have been obvious to the clinician in the office setting. The second meeting is mostly a discussion of the results of the testing, giving the patient and the family the most likely diagnosis, and recommending further treatment. Medical treatment at that time can include any one of the four FDA-approved medications. Also, at the second visit, an extensive discussion is entered into with the patient and their family members or caregivers regarding the stage of the disease and what to expect.

There are many ways of describing the stages of Alzheimer's disease. However, for the sake of simplicity, I will use mild, moderate, or severe when describing the stages to family members. In the mild stages, a patient is essentially forgetful. Based on the fact that they already have Alzheimer's disease, they will begin to neglect daily living activities. This can be as simple as forgetting to take medications or the ability to manage their financial affairs like they once did. In this stage, the patient is typically still very capable of living on their own but they do need a bit of assistance, and they need reminders in the form of phone calls or alarms to take the medications, or they may need some of the family members to watch them as they pay bills. In this stage, there may also be subtle changes in personality where the family may notice that the patient is more irritable than usual, many times ascribing this to "just getting older."

In the late-mild stages, a physician may begin to express concern about continuing to allow the patient to drive a vehicle. This is an enormous issue. First, the patient doesn't want to give up driving, and the family doesn't want the patient to stop driving either. The data regarding driving and when to stop the patient from driving with a dementing illness such as Alzheimer's is not very good. There is some data that suggests the clinical dementia rating scale (CDR) is helpful in this situation. This is one of the tests that a psychologist will probably administer. If that data points to the fact that the patient is unsafe, the psychologist or neurologist will usually ask the patient to voluntarily relinquish their license. If they do not agree to do so, the matter has to be turned over to the State. The State then determines whether or not the patient is safe to drive. To gain a better sense of the safety on the road, a physician will sometimes ask the family if they had a small child who was strapped into a car seat, would they feel safe with their family member driving that child around town alone. If the family member answers no, that is usually a fairly good indication that the patient is incapable of driving safely. Other indications that a patient needs to stop driving include accidents and moving violations over the past five years, the patient restricting their own driving to 60 miles per week or less, and new impulsive behaviors or road rage behind the wheel of the car. This is a very serious health issue given the advancing age of our population and the risk that impaired drivers can pose not only to themselves but also to others on the road.

By the moderate stages of Alzheimer's disease, the patient is beginning to have significant problems managing affairs at home. This may include difficulty in preparing even simple meals and significant behavioral changes where the patient begins to get very confused at the end of the day. The confusion at the end of the day is sometimes referred to as "sundowners." The patient may hallucinate rather significantly. These problems make it difficult if not impossible for them to live alone. Usually by this stage they require either a caregiver to be with them in the home or a move into an assisted living facility. The patient and family must determine what their collective preference is.

As the disease progresses through moderate stages and begins to approach the severe stage, it becomes obvious to even the most resistant family members that there is something wrong with the patient. Those closest to the patient will begin to notice that the patient has some difficulties with balance and walking. At this stage, they will also begin to notice difficulties with speech. The balance issues are typically mild if the patient does not have any other health issues that interfere with walking such as arthritis in the hip, nerve damage in the feet, spinal cord injury, strokes, etc. They may have the occasional sense of imbalance and a rare fall. Usually at this stage they can get past this with physical therapy, a home exercise program, and, occasionally, the use of a cane. However, if the patient has any issues that impair balance, they will frequently need an assistive device, such as a walker, to move around safely. Issues impairing balance may include arthritis in the weight bearing joints, peripheral neuropathy, or age related muscle atrophy. Remember, the wider the walker base, the better for the patient.

As the patient transitions from moderate to severe disease, their behavior can become more erratic and at times they will lash out at caregivers.

They begin to have more issues with sleep at night. These behavioral issues are very difficult to treat. The problem is that there are currently no FDA-approved medications for the treatment of behavioral issues in dementia patients. Initial treatment is to try the simplest nonpharmacological interventions. This may be as simple as setting a time at which the patient goes to bed and a time at which the patient gets up every day. It also proves helpful for the patient to go outside and see the sunshine without the filter of windows every day. It is preferable to do this towards the end of the day if possible. I encourage family members to have the patient exercise as this may improve sleep quality as well. Understandably, many of these things may not be possible with the patient; however, I still think it is worth trying as the benefits may be significant and the risk is minimal.

Over the years, many medications have been looked at for the treatment of agitation in Alzheimer's patients and, unfortunately, no medication has proven to be superb. Medications tried have included selective serotonin reuptake inhibitors such as Prozac and Zoloft, anticonvulsant medications such as Lamotrigine and Depakote. Also, medications such as benzodiazepines like Valium and Ativan have been studied, and finally antipsychotics have been looked at. Each group of medications has its pluses and minuses, and some of these medications carry more risk than others. Determining which one to try is based on numerous things including the physician's preference, other medications the patient is taking, and the family's preference of risk tolerance. Some of these medications carry with them a black box warning - meaning the drug can increase the risk of death. Once the patient is into the advanced stages of the disease, it is my belief that the physician's goals are to try and keep the patient as comfortable and happy as possible by encouraging the patient to be in a routine, stable, and pleasant environment.

Many times, once the patient enters the severe stages of the disease, their needs will exceed even the most attentive family's abilities. As a result, someone must be brought into the home to assist the family in caring for the patient. These tasks may include bathing, changing diapers, changing soiled linens, doing laundry, etc. Just as importantly, discussions must be entered into with the family, particularly if they are considering assisted dementia care in a facility. Whenever this transition occurs, many times the family is fraught with guilt over having to institutionalize their family member. Psychological support services are often recommended at this point for everyone involved. It must be pointed out to family members that if the patient stays in their home and something happens, the guilt will be even more intense.

Ultimately, the patient loses the ability to walk safely and to talk coherently. Death is usually near at this point. Common things that cause the demise of these patients include infections such as pneumonia, urinary tract infections, and skin infections. The less ambulatory the patient, the more likely the infections. When a person is bedbound, they are at higher risk of infections due to skin breakdown. Also, in the recumbent position there is greater difficulty coughing forcefully and the patient becomes unable to clear secretions from their lungs making them susceptible to pneumonia. Nutritional issues also become more prominent at this stage as the patient may have a very poor appetite and will begin to suddenly lose weight. The patient may also lose the ability to swallow. It has been documented in the literature that older patients who are slightly underweight have a higher risk of death if they become ill.

In the end, the disease is psychologically harder on the survivors than it is on the patient. The survivor's transition to life without that family member is made easier through good interaction with the physician and strong psychological support with family and friends.

Dr. William Justiz
Naples, Florida

Dayna note: Willie, my brother-in-law, often tried to tell me something was wrong, that something was beginning with Mom's brain. Even though he meant well *and* was a leading neurologist, it 'went in one ear and out the other' as Mom used to say. Looking back, I wish we had gotten her tested much earlier and had known. There are many plans we could have made and things we could have done during earlier stages of the disease.

Living Arrangements: Alane Roberts

I loved Sunday afternoons at my Aunt Edith's house — except for one thing: going to the "old folk's home" every single Sunday evening before church. It was a ritual she never missed, and I dreaded it every time I spent a Sunday with her — that gnawing ache in my gut about 4:30 p.m. when she called us in from our play to get cleaned up.

A sprawling, ugly, one-story monstrosity, the nursing home was painted a ghastly green inside, and was smelly and dreary and clinical, and I truly hated everything about it as a child. The people in it scared me, too.

These images are often dreaded recollections of an aging senior when they beg their children to never "put them in a home." Children are often plagued with guilt because they have promised that they never would, and yet life is making it very difficult to keep that pact. Blessedly, the options for care for an aging loved one are very different today than the frightening and odd-smelling places of the past.

As with any other part of the aging process, I recommend using an expert when looking for a home or facility for your loved one. Online searches can tell you where a facility is located, and how much it will cost, but an experienced advisor will ask you questions and learn about the story of the senior, helping you with recommendations that suit the whole person, not just their personal care needs.

Matching a care facility to a senior involves more than a zip code and a dollar amount. It involves connection to a sense of community, cultural fit, activities, social interaction, and the 24/7 that your loved one will be in an environment.

The option that best suits your loved one and their needs truly depend on where they are in the aging process when you reach out for help. I strongly advise every family to have a conversation about caring for the older members of the family while everyone is happy and healthy and can still pull up their own pants. Nothing is more trying and traumatic than trying to make decisions in the midst of a catastrophic event, when emotions are high, nerves are frayed, and money is tight. Truly, one of the most wonderful gifts a parent can give a child is to plan ahead for their care, and make their wishes known.

The best-kept secret in the aging process is the first place on the place-ment journey — independent living. These communities are similar to apartment complexes, but offer dining and food services, and a plethora of activities and community outings. This "first step" kind of placement is ideal for the active senior who is often alone and isolated. I highly recommend that aging seniors consider independent living prior to an illness or accident, to keep them active and connected to a sense of com-munity. An independent living community, while it offers no services it-self, is usually contracted with a personal assistance services company, in order to provide services for assistance when the senior begins to need a little help with activities of daily living. Using the Greater Houston area as an example, costs for independent living begin at about $1,600 a month and can be as high as $6,000, depending on the location, and amount of services that are used.

Assisted living facilities are the next space in the placement continuum. When a senior needs help several times a day, an assisted living environ-ment is the answer. An assisted living facility offers a long-term care solution that combines housing, meal service, support care options, and health care support as needed. Assisted living provides caregiver support around the clock. Each assisted living community decides what level of care and support they will provide. Most communities offer levels of care in addition to the housing portion, and additional care can be added as needed when a senior's physical condition deteriorates. Services range from medication management and meal reminders to full support.

Another assisted living option is the residential care home, or personal care home. These are residences that have been remodeled to accommodate the needs of seniors, such as wheelchair access and roll in showers, and have been licensed by the state as a small assisted living. Residential care homes are ideal for the aging senior that needs a lot of hands on care. In many cases, the care home is a more economical option as well, particularly if the care need is high.

While all assisted living communities offer the same basic features of care and support, their look and 'flavor' can be very different. Some are modern, upscale, and offer more activities or amenities. Others are more relaxed and casual. A skilled advisor can guide you toward a community that suits the lifestyle to which your loved one is accustomed. Families can expect to pay $2,700 to $8,000 for assisted living based on the location and amenities of the facility, and the care needs of their loved one.

Memory care facilities are those that care for seniors suffering with Alzheimer's disease or dementia. Many assisted living communities have a special unit just for memory care residents, but there are also facilities that specialize in this particular issue. Memory care is the most expensive kind of assisted living, because they offer total support, not only assistance. Working with seniors with cognitive issues takes special training and support, in order to redirect, manage agitation, calm, and soothe frustrations for those in the midst of the progression of disease.

Many memory care communities require everyone on staff to receive special training so that they are equipped for any encounter with a memory care resident. Memory care costs can range from $3,500 to $9,000 a month.

Finding the care that a senior needs is a loving choice. It allows a caregiver to handle the care, while you enjoy the relationship with your loved one again.

Alane Roberts
ElderCare Advisor/President
Assisted Living Locators Houston
alane@assistedlivinglocators.com
www.assistedlivinglocatorshouston.com

Dayna note: Someone who followed me on Facebook suggested I speak with Alane. I didn't even know this sort of service existed and wish I had known this at the beginning of the process. If I had, we might not have had to move quite so much as Mom deteriorated.

THE LAWYER: MICHAEL HOLLAND

ELDER LAW ATTORNEYS help families deal with issues specific to an aging population and these issues are only going to increase as time passes. We help families that are sometimes desperate for help. Let me illustrate with an example of the type of problems Elder Law Attorneys deal with every day:

Bill and Sara called the firm with concerns about Sara's mother who was suffering from Alzheimer's. Her disease had progressed to the point where Sara could no longer care for her mother. She tried to take care of her mother at home with the help of her husband, but Sara was exhausted, frustrated and had little time for herself or her own family. They had looked into nursing home care for her but they could not afford to pay the $5,000 per month fee for the nursing home. That would have quickly depleted their entire life's savings. They did a little research online and discovered a Medicaid program that offered assistance in these kinds of circumstances. They had several obstacles however, because Sara's mother had monthly income exceeding the amount allowed to participate in the program. Bill and Sara had been laying awake at night worrying about how they would ever get out of this dilemma.

Luckily, Bill had a friend that suggested they contact an Elder Law Attorney. Neither Bill nor Sara had ever heard of Elder Law Attorneys. That's not uncommon. A lot of folks are not aware that there is a small group of lawyers that focus on issues that elderly people face everyday.

Bill and Sara came into the office to discuss their options. Medical necessity was not an issue as Sara's mother was indeed suffering from Alzheimer's. The second hurdle to solving their problem was for us to prepare a Miller Trust (sometimes called a Qualified Income Trust) which solved the problem of Sara's mother having too much monthly income to qualify for help. While in the office, we discovered that Sara's mother had assets that exceed the countable resources that Medicaid allowed. Bill had heard that they could just "spend down" his mother-in-law's assets or give them away. Because we see this kind of mistake being made often, we were able to steer them away from the bad advice they had heard from friends in order to help them avoid costly delays in benefits.

The final issue was Sara's mother owned her own home and they heard that Medicaid would take her home. That was a valid concern but we also had a simple fix for that problem that preserved her home.

Elder Law Attorneys practice in very focused areas of the law and Bill and Sara's problems were not out of the ordinary. We were able to discuss the assets Sara's mother owned and how to best address each specific item in a way that allowed the family to get the best use of those assets, to preserve as much of them as possible for the future care of her mother and to obtain help with the soaring nursing home costs.

I asked Bill and Sara what they would like to see as the best outcome for Sara's mother. Their answer was to get the best possible care for her mother, to have her cared for in a place where she would be comfortable and safe and to preserve as much of her assets as possible so they could take care of her future needs. We aim to please and wanted to know what that would look like to the client.

The look of relief on Bill and Sara's faces when they left our office was noticeable. The most important concern that Sara had was that her mother be taken care of and we were able to accomplish that for her.

In my opinion, Elder Law is a very rewarding area of the law. I consider my clients to be the very best clients in the world. Why? Because they are trying everything they can to help someone they love who is in desperate need of help. In many instances, the family has tried to take care of their loved one on their own and they begin to feel the enormous burden that it puts on their time, emotions and resources. Elder Law Attorneys take an interest in the things that keep our clients awake at night. Their concerns become our concerns.

However, practicing Elder Law is sometimes an emotionally taxing experience because we see the raw emotions of clients as they scramble to meet the needs of their loved one as they continue their physical and mental decline. This is especially true when the loved one suffers from Alzheimer's.

As an Elder Law Firm we sometimes have to rally to help new clients when a crisis situation arises. Periodically we get a phone call from a frantic family member who advises that the hospital plans to release their loved one within 48 hours and they don't know where to take them or what to do — knowing they cannot provide the care themselves. That is where a good Elder Law Firm can provide guidance.

A good Elder Law Attorney can prepare many documents necessary for elderly clients, such as a Financial Durable Power of Attorney, Medical Power of Attorney, Physician Directives, HIPAA Medical Records Release Authorizations, Wills, Trusts, Organ Donor Designations and Power of Attorney Revocations to name just a few.

When an attorney says he or she "practices elder law" find out what types of matters the attorney normally handles. The key to finding the right lawyer for you is simple: engage an attorney who routinely addresses the types of problems that concern you. Many of our clients have issues with dementia and Alzheimer's. Many more have physical ailments that limit their mobility and interfere with basic life skills.

Just as most doctors are not skilled in every area of medicine, most attorneys are not skilled in every area of the law, especially the everyday facets of elder law. You want someone who is familiar enough with the problem you need solved to know how other aspects of the law might impact the steps you are considering.

As seniors age, they frequently find themselves dealing with complicated financial and health issues. Typical dilemmas involve retirement, end-of-life decisions, Social Security benefits, estate planning, long-term care, Medicare benefits, Medicaid coverage, nursing home care, and in-home health care. These get complicated. That's where the advice of a reliable Elder Law Attorney may help.

Elder Law Attorneys help seniors preserve their resources, protect their hard earned life savings from expensive costs of long-term care, and at some later point, guide families through the probate process. Getting competent legal direction makes the entire process smoother and provides the best possible final result for the elder and his or her family.

Look for an Elder Law Attorney who provides the following services:

- Advice on protecting assets to avoid impoverishing one spouse when the other needs nursing home care
- Filing for Medicaid assistance
- Long-term health matters

- Disability planning through financial and health care powers of attorney
- Incapacity planning through the use of living wills and living trusts
- Estate planning through the use of trusts, wills and other legal instruments
- Creation of necessary documents such as financial power of attorney, medical power of attorney, physicians directives, organ donation, and wills
- Probate and ways to avoid probate
- Questions about nursing home issues including patient rights and quality of care

I encourage clients to ask questions about the services to be provided. Attorneys should make themselves available to take client phone calls and to give them as much personal attention as they need. A good Elder Law Attorney explains the entire process from start to finish. It is important the client knows all about the process, which reduces the client's fear and anxiety. It is important to help the client with whatever concerns they have that are keeping them up at night. It is my opinion that if you do not have a lawyer that helps in this way, you've got the wrong lawyer.

Keep in mind that a good attorney keeps a full schedule. You may speak with a legal assistant when you first call to set the appointment. That assistant should be able to answer your questions or be able to get the answers for you quickly so you can decide if you want to schedule the appointment. But above all else, expect to be able to meet with the attorney. A good Elder Law Attorney should welcome your calls and questions.

Michael Holland
Holland Elder Law Firm
www.houstoneldercareattorneys.com

Dayna note: I used an attorney early on to help me navigate the Veterans Administration process for benefits Mom was entitled to. She may have been eligible early on for Medicaid but we did not realize that. An elder care attorney can guide you through the rules, the regulations, the mind numbing processes to get all this done. Again, looking back, something else I wish I had known.

Documents You Will Need: Nancy Rust

As OUR PARENTS age, our parents realize their needs and capabilities are changing. As children and caregivers, we want to be able to encourage and enable their independence to the greatest extent possible; allowing them to make their own decisions until it becomes necessary for someone to step in and either make relevant decisions or honor earlier wishes. Preparation is the key to making this process the easiest it can be for our parents, our families, and us. The largest part of preparation encompasses conversation and paperwork, with decisions and paperwork evolving and changing over time. The following are some forms that need to be considered, completed, and then revised as circumstances change:

Health Care Proxy Form (Medical Power of Attorney) — This document gives authority to someone you designate who will make health care decisions for you if you are unable. The person chosen should be someone you trust to carry out your wishes, which you have confirmed that he/she understands clearly. In choosing this person, you need to consider whether he or she is likely to have full use of his or her faculties when you need assistance. Spouses, friends are likely candidates, but they may not be able to speak for you when you need them most.

Durable Power of Attorney Form — This document gives someone the authority to take care of you financially if you are unable. As you are giving control of your money to someone else, this form should not be completed without serious consideration. The person you stipulate must be someone you trust to make financial decisions for you. With this form you are giving them the keys to your castle.

HIPAA Form — This gives the medical community the authority to share your medical information with whomever you have designated.

Directive to Physician Form (Living Will) — This spells out your wishes for your physician and loved ones. In both cases, you need to have a conversation confirming that your physician and loved ones understand and will honor your wishes.

Donor Registry Form — Complete this state form if you want to donate organs.

Last Will and Testament —This document guides your executor and family after you die and should be created by an attorney.

Nancy Rust
YCollaborative
www.YCollaborative.com (has a workbook for these documents and more)

Dayna note: This was one area where we had already taken care of things and it saved us so much time and effort. Wills were already in place. When Dad started having strokes, long before we knew there was a problem with Mom, I insisted I have Powers of Attorney for both of them (legal and medical), last wishes, Directive to Physician forms, and co-signing privileges on all their bank accounts. One thing that did prove challenging was the US Social Security system — this government organization does not recognize a legal Power of Attorney. I had to go in person with Mom to a local Social Security office to get my name on her account and obtain the proper permissions to talk to Social Security moving forward on the phone. Other documents we needed during this adventure were a notarized Marriage Certificate from the courthouse and Dad's notarized discharge papers from the VA. The efficiency of the US government during these fun exercises will make you drink more wine than usual.

Long-Term Care Insurance: Honey Leveen

Insurance disclaimer: The following is based on the author's personal experiences and opinions.

Much of the legacy we leave may be measured by how honestly we've dealt with life's most painful truths. Often, such truths are the most obvious, yet hardest to see clearly.

I've specialized in long-term care insurance (LTCi) since 1990. That's a long time. I've seen a few hundred of my nearly 3,000 clients collect from policies I've sold them. This is just the tip of the iceberg, however; many more will need to collect from their LTCi as time goes on.

I see scenarios just like Dayna's play out again and again. For different reasons, when a parent needs LTC, family members who've always gotten along well may find themselves at odds with each other. It is exactly as Dayna describes. The absence of sufficient, readily available money to swiftly access long-term care (LTC) aggravates an already highly stressful situation.

People who own LTCi also commonly suffer familial dysfunction similar to Dayna's. What makes things so different for them is that their LTCi policies pay out significant, meaningful amounts of money when LTC is needed. This is often a huge game changer. LTCi tends to subdue the emotional discord Dayna describes. Relationships don't suffer as much, and outcomes are better. The money people collect from LTCi provides them with dignity, choices, access, and options they would not have otherwise had.

Sadly, most of us still do not own LTCi. Sadder still, it is too often well-educated people with good incomes and a whole lot to lose who choose to be unprepared for LTC.

Such people come up with what they think are fabulous excuses to avoid discussing what might happen to them at the end of their lives. There seems to be a disconnect between our intellect and our emotions when it comes to LTC planning.

According to www.longtermcare.gov and other reputable sources, at age 65, there's a 70 percent chance of needing LTC. These odds go up with each year we age. Visit Genworth's Cost of Care Calculator (find it in the Resources area of www.honeyleveen.com) to see just how expensive LTC is in your locale.

Most LTC in the US is provided on an unpaid basis, disproportionately by women, who often have to sacrifice their careers, savings, and relationships to provide care. LTC already costs American families dearly, yet the worst of this crisis is yet to come.

First Lady Rosalynn Carter once said, "There are only four kinds of people in this world: those who have been caregivers, those who are caregivers, those who will be caregivers, and those who will need caregivers."

Here are some simple responses to major misconceptions about LTC and LTCi. More complex answers are found on www.honeyleveen.com or by calling me, at no obligation:

LTCi is too expensive. Not true. What may be expensive is needing LTC for anything but a short time and not owning LTCi. Policyholders usually collect back all premiums they've paid over the life of their policy in a few short months. Premiums are customized for each person and can be made to fit into almost anyone's budget.

The government pays for LTC. The type of LTC the government pays for is not what you would freely choose.

Medicare covers LTC. No it doesn't! Medicare covers acute medical problems and a restrictive, conditional amount of home or in-patient rehabilitative care that most people don't qualify for.

The LTCi industry is threatened. It's true that the number of carriers selling LTCi has shrunk; there are valid reasons. Policyholders are not in danger. LTCi carriers remain staunchly committed to the market. They realize the LTC crisis and oncoming Senior Tsunami isn't going away any time soon, and are in it for the long run.

LTCi only pays for nursing homes. The opposite is true. The great majority of LTCi policies pay comprehensively, for care at home, in adult day care, assisted living, and nursing homes. They enable you to increase the odds you will not need LTC provided in a nursing home.

Here are some of many silly excuses smart people give me to avoid conversing about LTCi while they're healthy and can find reasonable premiums:

My wife will take care of me. Really? Your wife will be eager and physically capable of helping you bathe and dress, for example? You don't mind the thought of her last memories being about the physical, emotional, and financial burdens of caring for you?

That won't happen to me. Really?

My kids will take care of me. Really?

I'll kill myself. Really?

I can't afford LTCi. Many people claim LTCi is too expensive, despite the fact that we tailor LTCi premiums to fit into most people's budgets. Situations like this one happen frequently: an acquaintance tells me she can't afford LTCi premiums. This person's mother needed LTC for an extended length of time, at great sacrifice to the family. A week later this person announces she is making a two-week trip to Mt. Everest Base Camp/African photo safari/Tahiti or another exotic locale, or is buying a top-of-the-line car/kayak/audio equipment, etc. She has the money to do that but can't afford LTC premiums. Where's the disconnect?

Here's another common scenario: I get incoming calls with Caller ID stating: METHODIST HOSP RE-HAB. The caller is the daughter or son of someone who's just broken their hip or suffered a stroke. They ask me to come sell their parent LTCi. I have the unpleasant task of trying to tactfully explain that their parent is uninsurable. Sometimes the child is incensed by this news. I suggest the child is of ideal age to find reasonably priced LTCi for themselves; this might be a wise idea if they want to assure a similar scenario doesn't play out when at the end of their lives. The child is normally not interested. The reason is that the family is in the worst kind of turmoil, duress, and dysfunction. They are scurrying around trying to cobble together LTC for their parent, and there isn't sufficient, readily accessible money to pay for it. This is the scenario Dayna and I urge you to avoid by doing reasonable, responsible LTC planning, now.

What all of my LTCi clients have in common, regardless of their incomes, is the ability to honestly, openly discuss LTC in advance. Most of my clients have had firsthand experiences similar to Dayna's. They've learned from them, and taken action to avoid the consequences of not being prepared for their own long-term care.

Honey Leveen
Long-Term Care Insurance Specialist
www.honeyleveen.com

Dayna note: I saw Honey speak at a meeting several years ago and immediately came home and told Wonder Husband all I had learned. We had watched his family, his ex-wife's family, and now, my family struggle to make ends meet once they had to start paying for care for elderly parents. Charlie and I signed up immediately for the best plan available. We are secure knowing that when the time comes, our kids will not have to pay anything out of pocket for our care. It is covered. Mom had very little savings and no care plan or insurance in place. We paid thousands of dollars out of our savings to keep Mom safe and cared for — many people don't have that luxury. Learn more about long term care insurance now — don't put it off any longer.

THE CAREGIVERS AND THEIR CAREGIVERS SPEAK

THE CAREGIVER OF an Alzheimer's patient ends up needing caregivers as well – a spouse, a partner, children, other immediate family members, friends, neighbors, and more. Many will want to help but do not know what to do or how to handle what is happening to the caregiver. It is important if you are the caregiver of a caregiver that you know how hard this will be on you. You will be dealing with mood swings, anger, depression, and tears. If you have kids, they will be at a loss on what they are supposed to be doing. The time-consuming efforts will often take the caregiver away from you – physically and mentally. Your marriage or other relationships will be tested and strained. In order to make it to the other side of this journey, here are what caregivers and their caregivers recommended when asked on Facebook:

- It was so very hard to watch your journey, knowing there was no way to help prepare you for what you were going to experience. It's a solitary journey. Maybe that's what others should know... how wholly alone the caregiver can feel in the experience.

- For those who are full-time, hands-on caregivers to someone living with us, every now and then someone would ask, "Is there anything I can do for you?" and I wouldn't be able to think of what that might be. I was so overloaded with decision making that I couldn't even think. The biggest help that came my way were the people who offered something specific like, "Can I bring you all dinner one night next week?" or "Is there a time when I could sit with your Mom for an hour or so to give you a break?" That was a huge help.

- No matter how many times my wife asked what I thought we should do, I always deferred to her, it was her Dad. I knew early on he needed to go to a facility but there was no way I could be the one to force it. It was awful for months on me and on the kids. When she finally admitted it had to be done, I didn't say, "I know." I said, "Whatever you want to do, I am here to help you."

- My sister was the primary caregiver and power of attorney. I know there were times she wished it wasn't her but she wouldn't back down. She tells me she wishes we could have all had more time with mom. My sister is the strongest most balanced person I know. She would let me know when she needed a break. We are lucky that mom raised us that way. We all came full circle in the end.

- What do you do when the caregiver refuses help? My mother-in-law takes care of her husband. We offer help but she refuses it. She does it all and refuses to talk about it but is trapped and locked (so he won't wander) in her home with her husband. He demands her attention full-time. She is strong willed and deflects all offers not of her own idea. We are scared to force the help on her.

- We came up with a plan that has family members call to say, "I am shopping nearby. What can I pick up for you and drop off while I am here in the area?"

- I needed my family to be more understanding of what I had to go through. They would come over and visit for an hour or so and never saw all the things I had to go through - bathing her, changing her diaper, making sure she took her meds, that she didn't fall. Instead, they would come over and complain if she had an odor or had a stain on her gown. Not one ever offered to stay over for a night and experience what had became routine for me.

- I wish other family members who were so full of excuses about why they could not take time out to help would have understood the impact of that--not only on me, but on our grandmother, who could not comprehend why they wouldn't even bother to visit for the last four years of her life. I know they lived across town (20 minutes is not that far), and I know they had jobs, but just a phone call to her or a one-hour weekend visit would have gone so far to help her morale. Even if they had stopped by to relieve me for a couple of hours every three months, that would have been miraculous. But they never did.

- My own husband was extremely supportive, and he would often do my mother's grocery shopping, pay her bills, and get her prescriptions so that I wouldn't have to expend that energy. He was also available to come help me so many times when she tried to get up out of bed or her chair by herself and would fall on the floor. As much weight as she lost, it was still difficult to lift her by myself, so I had to call on him to come over and help. Spouses of primary caregivers can't always give that much, but even if they can offer a supportive shoulder to cry on and listen as we vent about the difficulties of our day--that means so much.

- The only advice I have for a caregiver is to care for yourself during that time and have someone who you can crumble on because the caregiver is always expected to be strong and seldom do we feel we can leave that role because we feel we are out there for a reason. But the caregiver too, must be human.

- My brother and I did not have a close emotional relationship with our mom. As her primary caregivers during her Alzheimer's journey, we made sure she was well cared for; it was our duty and we would like to think we did it well. Because we weren't as emotionally invested in the relationship as those with close emotional ties with their Alzheimer's patient, it was probably easier on us. It still was a drain on time and finances and it required more focus from us so other parts or our lives lost our attention, but we didn't grieve an emotional loss. That is until about midway through her journey when we realized the enormous amount of fear our mother experienced every waking moment. Fear of the unknown, fear of not knowing, it was in her eyes, in her words, in her motions, it was ever-present. As distant a mother as she was - she protected us from fear. Realizing she would experience fear nearly every day of her remaining life and we couldn't make it go away was the worst part of the journey as her caregivers.

• It's not so much what I wish they had known to do, it's what more I wish I could have done to communicate to them. As much as I talked about the challenges we faced and people seemed to really listen, I could tell they never really understood. They couldn't. Not until they were there, in the moment themselves. And I did grieve for them. I tried so hard to communicate the insidious nature of this disease, to help prepare my friends, to communicate what I had painfully learned. But I knew they were outside the bubble and would remain there. Because who in their right mind would want to venture into that bubble if they didn't have to?

• Just adding this observation as both a caregiver and wife of a caregiver, at separate instances. All the spare time was very surreal after our loved one's passing. Life had become so much hospital; our social network was doctors and nurses. We actually had to figure out how to integrate back into living. No one could remember what we used to do before all the medical stuff happened. I wasn't prepared for that.

- I do it all and rarely ask for help. The worst part for me was when I would finally ask for help and it fell upon deaf ears. I will dance over flaming glass to give my parents the care they need. They did for it for me but the lack of help from my brothers and sisters adds to my moodiness, my bitterness. I feel imprisoned.

- The decision to move my mom was made by my two older brothers. I knew it was the right decision for our family, but I fought it every way I knew how. She was very angry with me that day, since I was the one to take her there. I was overcome with guilt and sadness. I felt like I had let her down (and my father) for not being able to care for her myself. I also knew it was the beginning of the end, and soon she wouldn't know the difference if I came or went. My mom existed for another 3 years. And, my brothers who had made the original decision rarely helped or came to visit. It was sad.

- The hardest part is the utter emotional exhaustion of dealing with my mom's confusion, anger, and suspicion (she hides her purse or sleeps with it) and the painful responsibility of making decisions for her "behind her back" because she doesn't realize she has dementia. It's heartbreaking to watch the mental decline. And personally, my friendships are failing because I can't get away on evenings or weekends to get together. I feel guilty going to dinner and a movie with my hubby because it costs $80 for the caregiver yet I am trying desperately to save some part of our relationship, that time away is vital.

> Dayna note: This was the most difficult section to write and edit. I originally asked my husband and teenage son to write this section, to write about what it was like to live with me these three years, to take care of me, to try to figure out what mood I was going to be in at any minute. I know I personally feel like I lost three years of life with them. One night at dinner, my teenage son blurted out, "You cry all the time." As soon as he said that,

he felt horrible and tried to pretend he had said something else. That was the first time I saw how hard it was on him to be around me during all of this. It was hard on our marriage as well; there were arguments over things we would never have argued about in the past. And, my interest in sex was usually overshadowed by sadness or exhaustion. Wonder Husband really felt shunned. After several requests, both finally told me they just couldn't write this section, it was just too hard to put into words what this was like for them - it didn't seem right to complain or point out any of these hardships after what I had been through with Mom.

RECOMMENDED WEBSITES

THESE ARE THE websites most often suggested by friends and followers throughout these posts. For the latest suggestions we have received, visit www.yourdailysuccesstip.com/survivingalz.

Alzheimer's Association
www.alz.org

Hilarity for Charity
www.hilarityforcharity.org
Part of the proceeds from this book will be donated here. The organization works in partnership with the Alzheimer's Association to fund research and provide grants for caregivers in need.

Caring.com
www.caring.com

Alzheimer's Foundation of America
www.alzfdn.org

Walk to End Alzheimer's
www.act.alz.org

Caregiver Action Network
www.caregiveraction.org

The Caregiver Space
www.thecaregiverspace.org

Alzheimer's Blog
www.blog.alz.org

Alzheimer's Speaks
www.alzheimersspeaks.com

Recommended Books

Just like the websites, these are the books that friends and followers recommended throughout this journey. Again, for the latest suggestions, see www.yourdailysuccesstip.com/survivingalz.

The 36 Hour Day: A Family Guide to Caring for People who have Alzheimer's Disease, Other Related Dementias, and Memory Loss
by Nancy L. Mace, Peter V. Rabins

Still Alice
by Lisa Genova
You may have seen the movie but we suggest you read the book as well. It is amazing and so much was left out in the film.

The Ghost Rider: Travels on the Healing Road
by Neil Peart

Aging with Grace: What the Nun Study Teaches Us About Living More Longer, Healthier, And More Meaningful Lives
by David Snowdon

Final Gifts: Understanding the Special Awareness, Needs, Communication of the Dying
by Maggie Callanan, Patricia Kelley

Loving Someone with Dementia: How to find Hope while Coping with Stress and Grief
by Pauline Boss

Being Mortal: Medicine and What Matters in the End
Atul Gawande

Untangling Alzheimer's
by Tam Cummings

Moonwalking With Einstein: The Art and Science of Remembering Everything
by Joshua Foer

The Talk: Family Questions

Here are important topics to discuss with your family members and other loved ones concerning health matters, documents, finances, and end of life issues. Not only should you know their answers but also you should have the answers to these questions for yourself saved where someone can find them. If you can't get someone to answer these questions in person, try sending a copy. You'll find a printable document to download at www.yourdailysuccesstip.com/survivingalz. These questions aren't just for your elders. These questions are for spouses, grown children, best friends – anyone you care about that you may end up taking care of and making decisions for in the future. Knowing the answers to these questions will free up an unbelievable amount of time, grief, and guilt for everyone involved.

- Where are important legal documents located? This includes all information pertaining to your will and estate including executor name or names, Durable Power of Attorney, Medical Power of Attorney, HIPPA, Living Will, DNR directives, etc. This also includes Social Security cards, birth certificates, marriage certificates, divorce papers, real estate documents, car titles, and anything else you can think of.

- If former military, what branch did you serve in, what dates, what was your discharge date and status, and where are your discharge papers?

- Do you have a safe deposit box? If so, where is it located and where is the key to access the box?

- Do you have a life insurance policy? If so, what is the company, account number, and contact information?

- Do you have medical insurance? If so, what is the account number and contact information?

- Do you have Long Term Health Care Insurance? If yes, what are the company, account number, and contact information?

- What are your bank accounts as well as mortgage, credit card, and investment accounts? Include company names, account numbers, and contact information.

- Where is a list of user IDs and passwords for all of your online accounts?

- Who are your current doctors and what is the contact information?

- What are your current prescriptions, dosage amounts, and, pharmacy contact numbers?

- How do we gain accessibility to your home including the keys and security code(s)?

- Who are your closest neighbors or friends that can be contacted in case of an emergency and what is their contact information?

- If you need care, do you prefer a nursing home, private care home, VA facility, or other? Have you already made any arrangements for continued care? If so, what is that information and where is any documentation?

- If your home needs to be sold, do you have any specific instructions?

- If you can no longer take care of your pet(s), what is the vet contact information and where would you like your pet(s) to go?

- Stop all the drugs and preventative measures, only giving medication for discomfort or pain, when I can no longer

  _____.

- Do you want a funeral, in a church, a party, or a wake? Do you have written instructions and if so, where are these instructions?

- Where will your final resting place be or where do you want your ashes scattered?

- What is your religious affiliation (if applicable) including where you worship and a contact name, and number?

- Do you want an obituary in a local and/or out of town paper? Have you written one already. If so, where is it? If not, what do you want in your obituary?

- Do you want flowers for services or donations made in your name to your favorite charitable organization?

- Are there specific persons you want notified upon your passing and what is their contact information including email addresses and phone numbers?

- If not included in a will, are there special items you wish to go to specific family members such as furniture, photos, keepsakes, memorabilia, and more?

- Name information and dates of all marriages and children you have had including divorce and death dates as well.

- Last, more for future family members more than anyone interview your loved one using the recording capability on your mobile device or computer.
    ° Where were you born?
    ° Tell me your earliest memory as a child.
    ° Where did you go to school?
    ° Who was your first love?
    ° Do you have any regrets?
    ° What was the best trip you ever took?
    ° What was your first job?
    ° The more you can ask and record, the more future generations will know about their family and past.

Dayna note: We were fortunate in that I had taken care of most of these questions prior to Mom's diagnosis. The one question I never asked was, "If you do need care, where do you want to live?" That would have also been the time to initiate the conversation that living with us was not going to be an option – I had to protect my health and well-being as well as my relationship with my husband and with my kids. Not knowing the answer to that question was the source of great guilt for me throughout the process and, probably will be for a long time to come.

10 Alzheimer's Warning Signs

- Memory changes that disrupt daily life
- Challenges in planning or solving problems
- Difficulty in completing familiar tasks at home, or at leisure
- Confusion with time or place
- Trouble understanding visual images and spatial relationships
- New problems with words or in speaking or writing
- Misplacing things and losing the ability to retrace steps
- Decreased or poor judgment
- Withdrawal from work or social activities
- Changes in mood and personality

*From the Alzheimer's Association website

One Final Story...

NEIGHBOR AND ARTIST Cheryl A. Evans has taken her golden retriever to see mom almost weekly for the past two years. Mom passed yesterday morning. Yesterday afternoon, Cheryl was window shopping in Santa Fe, New Mexico. There was a beautiful sculpture of a dog with angel wings in the window. Cheryl went inside the shop to find out more. The proprietor handed Cheryl a bio sheet about the artist. The artist's name? Fran Nicholson. My obsession with thank you notes was taught to me by my wonderful mom. Apparently she is still finding a way to write them...

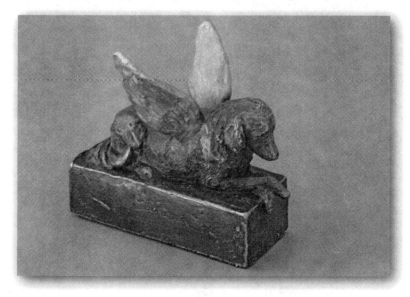

CPSIA information can be obtained
at www.ICGtesting.com
Printed in the USA
FSOW02n1146010916
24495FS